Clinical Handbook of
Weight Management

Clinical Handbook of Weight Management

Second Edition

Michael EJ Lean MA MD FRCP

Professor of Human Nutrition and Consultant Physician
Chair and Head of Department of Human Nutrition
University of Glasgow
Glasgow Royal Infirmary
UK

MARTIN DUNITZ

Although every effort has been made to ensure that the drug doses and other information are presented accurately in this publication, the ultimate responsibility rests with the prescribing physician. Neither the publishers nor the author can be held responsible for errors or for any other consequences arising from the use of information contained herein.

The opinions expressed in this book are those of the author and do not necessarily reflect those of Martin Dunitz Ltd.

© 1998, 2003 Martin Dunitz, an imprint of the Taylor & Francis Group

First published in the United Kingdom in 1998
by Martin Dunitz, an imprint of the Taylor & Francis Group,
11 New Fetter Lane, London EC4P 4EE

Tel.:   +44 (0) 20 7583 9855
Fax.:   +44 (0) 20 7842 2298
E-mail: info@dunitz.co.uk
Website: http://www.dunitz.co.uk

Second edition 2003

A CIP record for this book is available from the British Library.

ISBN 1-84184-104-8

Distributed in the USA by
Fulfilment Center
Taylor & Francis
10650 Tobben Drive
Independence, KY 41051, USA
Toll Free Tel.: +1 800 634 7064
E-mail: taylorandfrancis@thomsonlearning.com

Distributed in Canada by
Taylor & Francis
74 Rolark Drive
Scarborough, Ontario M1R 4G2, Canada
Toll Free Tel.: +1 877 226 2237
E-mail: tal_fran@istar.ca

Distributed in the rest of the world by
Thomson Publishing Services
Cheriton House
North Way
Andover, Hampshire SP10 5BE, UK
Tel.: +44 (0)1264 332424
E-mail: salesorder.tandf@thomsonpublishingservices.co.uk

Composition by Wearset Ltd, Boldon, Tyne and Wear
Printed and bound in Great Britain by The Cromwell Press, Trowbridge

Contents

Professor Michael EJ Lean MA MD FRCP holds the position of Chair and Head of Department of Human Nutrition at the University of Glasgow. He trained in medicine at the University of Cambridge and, after a brief spell as a junior heart surgeon in Edinburgh, concentrated on general medicine, diabetes and endocrinology. His clinical training was mainly in Aberdeen, but he returned to Cambridge to join the Medical Research Council and University of Cambridge Dunn Nutrition Unit. There he embarked on a research career in nutrition, specializing in diabetes, and in obesity and energy balance. In 1992 he was appointed to his present position, teaching and directing research into human nutrition, and its impact on many different aspects of health and medical practice. He has increasingly become involved in public health and health promotion measures to prevent disease, and to promote good health through healthy eating. In 1995 he was appointed a non-executive Director of the Health Education Board for Scotland. He has published over 100 peer-reviewed original papers, encompassing basic laboratory sciences, clinical research and clinical trials, nutritional epidemiology and health promotion. His work on obesity has been recognized as a winner of the André Mayer prize, co-authorship of clinical guidelines for diabetes and for obesity, including the influential Scottish Intercollegiate Guidelines Network (SIGN), and membership of advisory bodies for research councils and government departments.

Preface

During the training of doctors and nurses, the main focus has always been on the major killing diseases, and the major causes of pain and distress. The traditional goals of a medical training are to enable firstly a diagnosis to be made, secondly to interpret that diagnosis and give a prognosis or long-term outcome of the condition, and thirdly to offer treatment, when possible, with the aim of relieving suffering, curing a problem or improving the outcome.

Obesity has not, until very recently, featured strongly in medical training. There has been a widespread view that becoming overweight is a sign of a weak personality, a combination of gluttony and apparent sloth, very often accompanied by a degree of mendacity. A reluctance amongst medical practitioners to become involved in obesity and weight management has many contributory factors, clouded by the victim-blaming attitude which is now known to be inappropriate, on medical grounds, to convert a fat person into a thin one by way of inflicting a cure.

Recent years have seen a dramatic change in the needs of medical training towards prevention as a cornerstone of new health policies, and obesity is rapidly becoming recognized as one of the major correctable causes of ill health on a global scale.

The need to correct the trend of increasing obesity is one of the priorities of the National Health Services in the United Kingdom. Guidelines for clinical practice have been produced in a range of countries where the links between weight gain and a wide range of medical problems have been recognized. The problem is not restricted to the developed world. One of the curiosities of nutrition in the developing world is that obesity and its consequences tend to appear just as soon as malnutrition has been vanquished. Prevalence is already high and increasing rapidly in many developing countries.

In an average practice in a Western country, half of all adults will be overweight and between 10 and 25% in different countries will have reached the level of weight gain diagnosed as obese according to World Health Organization (WHO) criteria, based on body mass index (BMI), which virtually guarantees the development of symptoms and adverse effects on cardiovascular disease. A significant proportion of heart disease, and several major cancers (breast, uterus, prostate, colon) could be avoided, or at least delayed, if weight gain could be checked. Perhaps more importantly, the symptoms which lead overweight people to seek medical advice more frequently than normal-weight individuals could also be prevented. New research has improved the ability to diagnose, with waist circumference tending to replace the rather complex BMI, and current understanding of prognosis has improved with analysis of large epidemiological studies.

Recent advances have allowed the task of weight management to be made a little easier by recognizing that most of the benefits of weight loss can be achieved by losing *c.* 10 kg, and that this is achievable using a variety of different approaches. It is also now recognized that the main goal is probably not acute weight loss but rather maintenance of a stable body weight, resisting the tendency of appetites to exceed calorie needs for maintenance. This resetting of the goalposts has emerged from expert committees designing guidelines for best practice. The task now is to put effective guidelines into practice and to make them available, indeed market them, for people who have weight problems, and to try to engage them early in the process before they become very significantly overweight.

This second edition has been revised to provide an up-to-date background to obesity and an understanding of weight management for health professionals, and to offer outlines for management plans which can be instituted at a primary care level.

Michael EJ Lean

chapter 1

Introduction

There is a long history amongst parts of the health-care and medical professions of blindly attributing obesity to 'gluttony and sloth'. This classic victim-blaming attitude has been used to justify inactivity in medical management – *'It's your fault – pull yourself together! Exercise some restraint!'*. Overweight patients, who all have some underlying predisposition to weight gain, feel increasingly misunderstood, and this has compounded the distress caused by direct symptoms and major medical complications that they commonly suffer from.

All too often, doctors have ignored weight gain until it is very extreme, although they have been willing to treat secondary complications such as hypertension, hyperlipidaemia, non-insulin-dependent diabetes mellitus (NIDDM), arthritis or depression. From the point of view of the host of symptoms and of the secondary complications, there can be no doubt that obesity should be considered a disease, i.e. the process of extra weight gain should be considered a chronic disease process. The scientific and medical view of obesity is changing rapidly as its impact on health service is recognized, and also because of the rapidly growing evidence that adipose tissue is not just a repository for fat but is also the largest and most active endocrine organ in the body. At least 10 cytokine-related hormones are produced in adipose tissue and contribute to the diseases associated with obesity.

The World Health Organization (WHO) has recently reminded the medical world, and politicians, that obesity, with its genetic–lifestyle aetiology and catalogue of pathological consequences, is defined as a disease, coded internationally as ICD-10 E.66. The increasing prevalence of obesity and the huge burden of associated disease warrant use of the term epidemic. An increasingly educated public is beginning to demand a better service for weight problems, and doctors need to be able to provide appropriate understanding, treatment and support on a long-term basis, based on sound evidence for effectiveness.

The approach followed in this book is to address, in order, the epidemiology of obesity, its aetiology, the impact of obesity on health and health care, the evidence for benefit from weight management (including weight loss and long term maintenance) and then a number of interventions which can be employed in management.

Recognizing that the book may not be read from cover to cover, there is some repetition of key messages in different contexts. A number of references are included, especially for new or contentious issues, and some suggestions for further reading.

chapter 2

The scale of the problem

Definitions and criteria

By any criteria, around half of all adults in Western societies are now overweight and are liable to be encountering medical problems as a consequence. Because this figure has increased gradually, we have become accustomed to this increased fatness as part of the normal backdrop to our lives; however, most overweight people do recognize themselves as being fat and most make some conscious effort to control their weight problem. Surveys indicate that between 40 and 80% of adults take steps to restrict weight gain in the course of a year, and this behaviour can easily be identified in children from about the age of 10. However, the medical urgency is not yet widely recognized at a public health level. Doctors and other health professionals have also, to some extent grown accustomed to seeing more than half of all adults with elevated weights, and their significant associated health problems, as normality in their day-to-day working lives.

Most people make some efforts to control their weight at some stage in their lives. The proportion of adult people with a weight problem is >50%, perhaps >75%. As a crude simplification, about half of all adults have a visible weight problem in that they actually become overweight, but perhaps half of those (i.e. c. 25% of all adults) are actually able to control their weight to their reasonable satisfaction, albeit at a higher than ideal level. Of the 40–50% or so of all adults who never become overweight, perhaps half only achieve that by restrained eating, i.e. they have an underlying metabolic/genetic weight problem, but are able to control it. On this basis, *c.* 75% of all people probably have an underlying predisposition to become overweight but, in a Western environment, only *c.* 25% fail to control the problem *(Figure 1)*.

The English language contains many words used to denote fatness (e.g. stout, corpulent, obese, overweight, etc.) but there are few specific scientific terms or medical criteria to indicate this condition. Those used are definitions by convention, rather than diagnostic criteria directly related to pathology or clinical manifestations. The most widely used word in a clinical context, *obesity* derives from the Latin: *ob* = on account of, *esum* = having been eaten (from, *edere* = to eat). The term *obesity* does not indicate any specific diagnosis or pathological process. Referring to morbid obesity may sound as if it defines a specific diagnosis but it does not: *morbid* is another Latin work, meaning diseased.

Because people vary in stature, and this influences weight criteria for

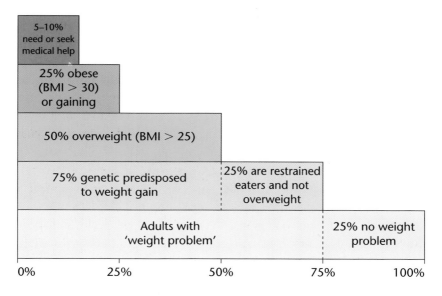

Figure 1 *Schematic presentation of proportions of the adult Western population with weight problems.*

being overweight or obese, height must be taken into account. This effect is in fact best corrected by height^2, and the degree of overweight is now defined, arbitrarily but by international convention set out in WHO guidelines, on the basis of body mass index (BMI): BMI = weight (kg)/height^2 (m^2). BMI is little influenced by height differences and relates reasonably closely to body fat content. It is accepted that other tissues also contribute to body mass and, for example, athletes will have a high BMI due to muscle mass. The acceptable, or normal, BMI range used to be 20–25 kg/m^2 but is now defined by the WHO as 18.5–25 kg/m^2. It straddles the acceptable average, previously known as the ideal body weight, at a BMI of *c.* 21 kg/m^2. This cut-off point was initially derived from life assurance tables to indicate the build with the statistically greatest life expectancy. It has more recently been shown to correspond well to the amount of body fat with greatest freedom from a large number of major diseases, and in a range of different populations. However, the variation between individuals in different populations is such that most health risks do not increase appreciably across a BMI range of 18.5–25 kg/m^2.

For epidemiological purposes, BMI $\geqslant$ 30 kg/m^2 has been defined as obesity, but it is important to recognize that this represents a late stage in the disease. Above a BMI of 30 kg/m^2 there are obvious increases in a wide range of medical consequences and it is almost impossible to exceed this BMI without a significant elevation of body fat. Obesity is a disease [International Classification of Disease (ICD) code E.66]: it is *the disease process of excess fat accumulation with multiple organ–specific pathological consequences.* This disease process incorporates components of excess or unregulated appetite, and an altered relationship between energy expenditure and body mass, representing the integration of a number of gene–nutrient interactions.

If health risk, or mortality ratio, is plotted versus BMI *(Figure 2)*, the curve is often described as being J-shaped. The sharply increased mortality in people with low BMI (a very small proportion of the total population) is now known to result largely from very thin smokers and others, especially older people, with subclinical diseases. When smokers are removed from the analysis, the curve tends to lose its J-shape

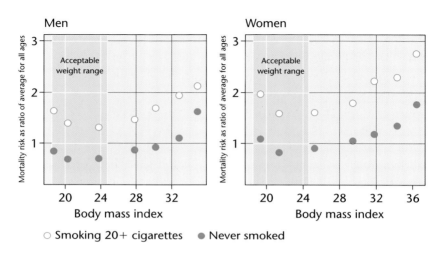

○ Smoking 20+ cigarettes   ● Never smoked

Figure 2 *Body weight, smoking and death rates for men and women.*
(Reproduced with permission from the Royal College of Physicians of London.[1])

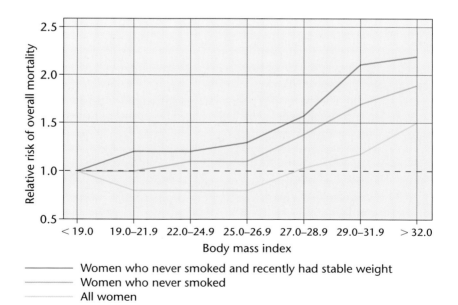

——— Women who never smoked and recently had stable weight
——— Women who never smoked
——— All women

Figure 3 *Relation between BMI and relative risk of overall mortality in women*
over 16 years. (Adapted from Manson et al.[2])

(Figure 3). In large studies, extreme thinness also increases mortality, but the adverse effects of obesity can be seen in both smokers and non-smokers *(Figure 2)*. Because such large numbers of people have a BMI >25 kg/m², and so few have a BMI <18.5 kg/m², the health hazards resulting from being overweight greatly outweigh those that result from extreme thinness in Western societies. The J-shaped curve is also flattened out in younger people *(Figure 4)*.

In older people, the mortality risk (mainly from cardiovascular disease) does not increase with BMI as markedly as in younger people. Indeed, above the age of 50, the right-hand side of the mortality curve is essentially flat above a BMI of 25 kg/m². This has sometimes been taken to mean that obesity is unimportant and that weight loss is of no value for older people. However, the greatest health hazards of being overweight amongst older people are not from aggravated cardiovascular disease, but rather from increased respiratory problems, arthritis, back pain, tiredness, depression, diabetes, etc., all of which demand medical attention. An acceptable range of BMI, i.e. 18.5–25 kg/m², can therefore

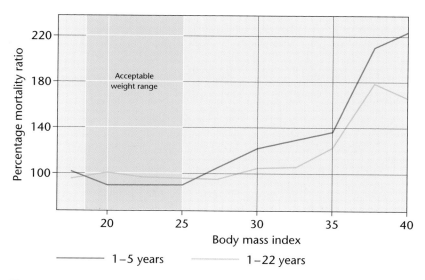

Figure 4 *Mortality ratio in relation to BMI in young men according to the length of their life assurance policies age 15–39. (Reproduced with permission from the Royal College of Physicians of London.[1])*

be applied for different reasons to adults of all ages, and weight management actually has a more immediate value to the overweight older patient. Moreover, weight loss in the elderly does still reduce cardiovascular risk factors, in a group where the total risk is, of course, much greater.

Recent years have seen a rapid rise in the proportion of people who are overweight in most Western countries and in urban communities in the developing world. Particularly worrying is the trend towards fatter children and adolescents. With this rise has come a predictable increase in obesity-related diseases and ill health in adults. Obesity rarely causes symptoms or secondary physical problems in childhood. However, it does contribute to psychological scarring, and a high likelihood of turning from overweight teenagers to obese adults. The rising prevalence of those who are overweight shows no sign of declining; therefore, doctors can expect further major increases in problems from this condition in the future *(Table 1; Figure 5)*. The economic cost of overweight and its complications are estimated at 8% of the total health

Table 1 Trends towards increasing obesity (BMI $\geqslant 30$ kg/m^2) in selected countries. (Reproduced with permission from Seidell et al[3] and Seidell and Flegal.[4])

Population	Year	Age (years)	Prevalence of obesity* (%)	
			Men	Women
England	1980	16–64	6.0	8.0
	1986/87		7.0	12.0
	1991		12.7	15.0
	1994		13.2	16.0
	1995		15.0	16.5
Finland	1978/79	20–75	10.0	10.0
	1985/87		12.0	10.0
	1991/93		14.0	11.0
The Netherlands	1987	20–59	6.0	8.5
	1988		6.3	7.6
	1989		6.2	7.4
	1990		7.4	9.0
	1991		7.5	8.8
	1992		7.5	9.3

Table 1 *Continued*

Population	Year	Age (years)	Prevalence of obesity* (%) Men	Women
	1993		7.1	9.1
	1994		8.8	9.4
	1995		8.4	8.3
Former East Germany	1985	25–65	13.7	22.2
	1989		13.4	20.6
	1992		20.5	26.8
Sweden	1980/81	16–84	4.9	8.7
	1988/89		5.3	9.1
USA	1960	20–74	10.0	15.0
	1973		11.6	16.1
	1978		12.0	14.8
	1991		19.7	24.7
Canada	1978	20–70	6.8	9.6
	1981	20–70	8.5	9.3
	1988	20–70	9.0	9.2
	1986/92	18–74	13.0	14.0
Brazil	1975	25–64	3.1	8.2
	1989		5.9	13.3
Japan	1976	20+	7.1	12.3
	1982		8.4	12.3
	1987		10.3	12.6
	1993		11.8	13.0
Japan	1976	20+	0.7	2.8
	1982		0.9	2.6
	1987		1.3	2.8
	1993		1.8	2.6
China	1989	20–45	1.7	4.3
	1991		2.9	4.3
China	1989	20–45	0.29	0.89
	1991		0.36	0.86
Western Samoa (urban)	1978	25–69	38.8	59.1
	1991		58.4	76.8
Western Samoa (rural)	1978	25–69	17.7	37.0
	1991		41.5	59.2

Obesity defined as BMI > 28.6 kg/m²

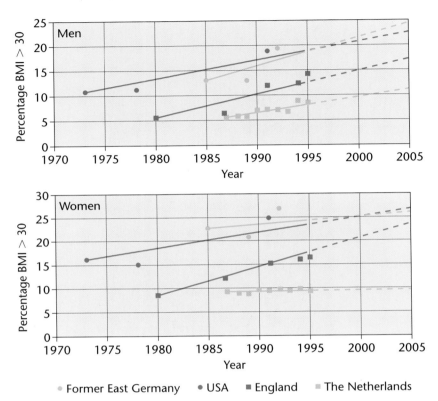

Figure 5 *Recent trends and projective rise in mortality risk with the consequence of weight gain.*

service budget in the USA. Slightly lower figures have emerged from analyses using different, perhaps more conservative, criteria in other countries. On the basis of studies in the UK and the Netherlands, the population-attributable risk from BMI > 30 kg/m^2 is *c.* 1% of total health service budgets in Western countries. Data on the extra costs of BMI of 25–30 kg/m^2 are difficult to obtain, but the total additional cost to health services from the large number of people who are overweight (or a crude estimate of the burden from the disease of obesity itself), is *c.* 4% of budgets *(Table 2)*. This is comparable with the total costs of other major diseases like cancers or diabetes. The cost of obesity in the USA is estimated at 7–8% of health care costs.

Table 2 Estimates of the economic costs of obesity.

Country	Year	Reference	Obesity definition	Estimated direct costs	National health care costs (%)
USA	1986	5	BMI > 29	US$39.3 billion	5.5
USA	1988		BMI > 29	US$44.6 billion	7.8
Australia	1989/90		BMI > 30	AU$464 million	>2
The Netherlands	1981–89	6	BMI > 25	1 billion guilders	4
			BMI > 30	250 million guilders	1
France	1992	7	BMI > 27		2
UK	1997	8	BMI > 30	£350 million	1

Fat distribution and waist circumference

The health hazards of obesity are compounded by the separate influence of central fat deposition. Excess fat on the abdomen (*a central fat distribution,* specifically with excess deep intraabdominal fat rather than just in subcutaneous sites) is a typical characteristic of men, compared with the more peripheral fat distribution of women. Central (intraabdominal) fat distribution is associated with a greater number of metabolic complications (including NIDDM, hypertension, hyperlipidaemia, heart disease and stroke) than extra fat that is principally in subcutaneous sites, i.e. on the legs or hips. The metabolic complications of a central fat distribution (***Tables 3a and b***) are linked to insulin resistance and a relative excess of adrenal steroids. The mechanism probably results from exposure of the liver to excessive release of fatty acids from an expanded

Table 3a Diseases and metabolic abnormalities related to obesity. (Amended from Seidell et al.[3])

Documented in well-controlled prospective studies	*Documented in cross-sectional or less well-controlled prospective studies*
Diseases	**Diseases**
Hypertriglyceridaemia, hyperuricaemia, hyperinsulinaemia, glucose intolerance	Gall bladder disease
	Kidney stones
	Breast cancer (after menopause)
Coronary heart disease and congestive heart failure	Menstrual abnormalities (long cycles, irregular menses, hirsutism)
Diabetes mellitus type 2	Pulmonary and respiratory diseases (e.g. sleep apnoea)
Gout	Renal disease
Arthrosis (osteoarthritis)	Skin complications
Degenerative joint disease	Anaesthesia and surgical procedures
Hypertension	Psychological problems (including impairment of self-image)
Endometrial carcinoma	Haemorrhoids
Varicose veins (women)	Non-alcoholic steatohepatitis (NASH)

Table 3b Conditions associated (as cause or consequence) with an abdominal fat distribution. (Adapted from Seidell et al.[3])

Men	Women
Prospective	**Prospective**
Ischaemic heart disease	Myocardial infarction and angina pectoris
Diabetes mellitus type 2	Diabetes mellitus type 2
Stroke	Stroke
	Endometrial cancer
Cross-sectional	**Cross-sectional**
Hypertension	Hirsutism and menstrual abnormalities
Arthrosis	Cushing's Syndrome
Peptic ulcer	Gall bladder disease
Sleep apnoea syndrome	Polycystic ovaries
Non-alcoholic steatohepatitis	Werner's syndrome
(NASH)	Familial partial lipodystrophy
	Psychosocial problems

Note: Unclear associations: gout, renal calculus
Abdominal obesity is associated with a lower risk of varicose veins

intraabdominal fat mass, as fatty acids impair insulin function on hepatocytes. It is important to recognize that the disease associations of central fat are present even in people who are not overweight, so the term central obesity is misleading.

A central fat distribution, with these disease predispositions, appears to be mainly under genetic control and the risks apply independently of total fatness based on BMI. On the other hand, fat distribution may also reflect nutritional status in early life. Intrauterine development or programming associated with low birth weight tends to lead to central fat accumulation. Fat distribution is also influenced by physical activity and weight loss (reducing central fat), and by physical inactivity, weight gain, smoking and excess alcohol (increasing central fat).

In a research setting, the amount of central fat can be measured by magnetic resonance imaging (MRI) or computerized tomography (CT) scanning, but the simple waist circumference measurement gives a very reasonable estimate. In the past, the waist/hip ratio was used, but this is being replaced with the simpler and more reliable waist circumference measurement as an indicator of risk. Hip circumference is affected by muscle mass as well as by fat. Excess intraabdominal fat, termed apple-shaped, or central or android fat distribution, marks the polymetabolic syndrome (***Table 3c***), insulin resistance, impaired glucose tolerance, NIDDM, adverse lipoprotein profiles and hypertension, and compounds the hazards of being overweight. People who are both overweight and have central fat distribution are at greatest risk of cardiovascular diseases and diabetes. Since both high BMI and central fat distribution contribute to a high waist circumference, this rather simple measurement offers a surprisingly powerful way to identify people in need of weight management. Waist measurement is more accessible to patients and health professionals alike than BMI for diagnosis and monitoring, with less opportunity for errors, and gives a more powerful prediction of health risk because it takes account of fat distribution as well as total fatness. Waist circumference, measured with a tape measure at a level

Table 3c Syndrome X or the polymetabolic syndrome associated with central fat distribution

• Glucose intolerance/diabetes	Insulin resistance
• Arterial hypertension	Hyperinsulinaemia
• Low HDL-cholesterol	Visceral obesity
• Hypertriglyceridaemia	Athero-thrombosclerosis
• Disturbances in haemorheology/haemostasis	Coronary heart disease
• Fibrinolytic abnormalities	Premature death

midway between the lowest ribs and the hip bone, (***Figure 6***) should ideally not exceed 80 cm (32 in) for women or 94 cm (37 in) for men. Below these figures, there is no need for weight loss. Above these levels, health problems are likely to develop with age either because of increasing BMI or because of a central fat distribution. If the waist circumference of a woman reaches 88 cm (35 in) or that of a man reaches 102 cm (40 in) then there is a serious problem (corresponding to BMI > 30 kg/m^2 or marked central fat deposition), and weight loss should be recommended. Waist circumference, perhaps surprisingly, is independent of height, so short and tall people have more or less the same waist (***Figure 7***). The cut-off points described above are now being used in health

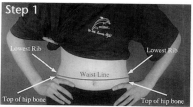

Find your natural waist line between your lowest ribs and your hip bones (by placing your hands on your hips)

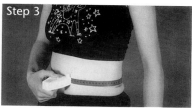

Relax your tummy by breathing out gently, and do not tuck it in. Press the button to fit the tape around your waist line. Adjust the tape so that it is level all the way round your waist

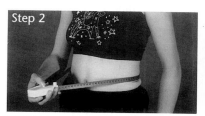

Place the tape around the waist line and insert the toggle into the slot

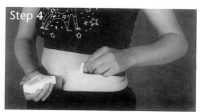

Take your thumb away from the button. Lift the toggle out of the machine. Be careful not to touch the button while removing the tape from your waist.

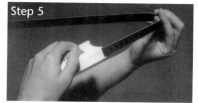

Read the number and the colour on the tape and record it on the form.

Figure 6 *How to measure waist circumference.*

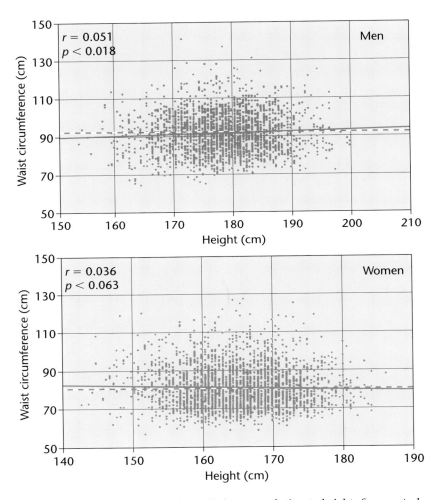

Figure 7 *Waist circumference bears little or no relation to height, from a study of 2183 men and 2698 women. (Reproduced with permission from Han et al.[6])*

promotion as 'action levels' to increase awareness of the need for weight management in countries across the world, although the absolute health risks for a given waist circumference do vary between populations.

A medical or a cosmetic problem?

There are some societies – e.g. African, Gypsy and others in antiquity – where being plump or fat has been considered attractive or desirable, as a sign of success or affluence. Where there was once widespread under-nourishment, or frequent famines, being a little overweight had survival value. It marked power or dominance in men, and greater fecundity and fertility in women. However, in most Westernized societies, being over-weight is viewed as unattractive, especially amongst women. Overweight people look older, and are often considered by both peers and the medical establishment to lack self-control. In surveys the words 'lazy', 'stupid' and 'unreliable' are often linked to obesity, and these attributes form the basis of opinion from both the general public and health pro-fessionals. In the UK, only 4% of doctors have a BMI $>30 \text{ kg/m}^2$, com-pared to *c.* 20% of their patients, so an attitude of victim blaming is perhaps not surprising.

The fashion and slimming industries have set up ideals of body shape that are at the low end of, and occasionally below, the acceptable range of BMI, using models with a prepubertal body morphology. These powerful media images have undoubtedly shaped unrealistic expecta-tions of 'ideal' weight for many people. For most people who are over-weight and who seek help, the driving force is more likely to be the immediate perception of their unattractiveness, even revulsion and depression at their shape, rather than a long-term concern for physical health. This has often been considered to present a problem for health professionals. It can be tempting to treat, in acquiescence to patients' cosmetic aims, believing (probably rightly) that health gain will proceed from weight loss whatever its primary intention. This approach can be criticized as being part of an unwanted medicalization of modern life. A frequently expressed alternative view is that medical services are not simply provided to solve cosmetic issues and that unless the patient rec-ognizes and complains about the medical consequences of being over-weight, treatment will not be offered. This harsh view is, to some extent, justified by results. The fashion and slimming industries have rather consistently promoted quick-fix slimming cures, claiming easy, dramatic

and rapid weight loss, with little emphasis on long-term weight maintenance that is essential for improved health. If patient and doctor set out
with radically different aims and belief systems, successful weight loss
and maintenance is unlikely.

It may be possible to bring the aims of the patient and the health professional together over the cosmetic issue by recognizing the concerns of
the cosmetically-challenged patient as impairing their quality of life,
and potentially contributing to later depression. The most frequent
reason given by people who join slimming clubs is 'to feel better'. The
goals of weight loss are rarely purely cosmetic, although the expecta-
tions of patients are influenced by a cosmetically-oriented lay literature,
which often leads to inappropriate expectations of what is possible. A
responsible and sympathetic medical service needs to explain the speed
and extent of weight loss that is actually possible by any method
(including those of commercial-organizations), and to emphasize the
need for an organized and well-supported approach to avoid weight
regain in the long term. Ultimately, obese people will not go to doctors
for help unless their expectation is of a sympathetic and informed professional who can do something to help.

chapter 3

The causes of weight gain, and patterns of weight change in different communities and individuals

The aetiology of obesity is often simplified, at a mechanistic level, into three components that govern energy balance: *diet, exercise* and *genes*. Attempts to identify a single cause within this triad will inevitably fail because all three must apply in every case. A failure in just one component would allow compensation from the others. Thus, in very simple terms, in populations with food provisions in excess of requirements, with high-fat diets (>30% of daily calories from fat) and without the need for physical exertion to obtain food, many people will gain body fat gradually throughout adulthood. However, not every individual becomes obese because genetic differences modify metabolism and appetite, and the individual is able to exert will power or self-restraint.

These factors all interact so that a high-fat diet (generally, also a low carbohydrate one) is particularly fattening for individuals with a genetic susceptibility to gain weight. In 1967, Jean Mayer[5] proposed that with very low physical activity and for people in sedentary jobs, appetite increases paradoxically to promote obesity – what is now termed the couch-potato effect. The same effect has been shown rather clearly in experimental animals. Appetite usually matches physical activity to keep weight steady. Rats can be made to exercise up to 6 hours daily and their weights remain unchanged. With very low levels of exercise, e.g. < 1 hour/day, the regulation between appetite and calorie requirement is lost, food intake actually increases and the animals put on weight. There is some evidence in humans that high-fat intakes are particularly fattening in sedentary individuals. It also seems that obese people, even if they feel exhausted by physical activity, are exercising well below the level needed to regulate appetite. Modest exercise by obese people actually *reduces* appetite, but the effort required (e.g. to walk briskly for 20 min) can be too great without training.

Why we eat what we eat

The physiological regulation of eating is complicated. Many factors contribute simultaneously, and they are somehow regulated to keep food intake within 1% of need over 50 years, for most of us.

Conventionally, we eat in response to appetite, which can be defined as a stage which moves us to seek food. If we fail to eat at that stage, hunger may develop – characterized by physical abdominal symptoms, and a need to hunt, steal, or fight for food.

Eating, introduces a pleasant feeling of fullness, known as 'satiety'. When we have eaten enough, satiety takes over for a variable period, usually 2–4 hours, before appetite re-emerges.

A great deal is known about the biochemical and neuroendocrine factors which affect appetite, (*Figure 8*), but most of us only occasionally develop a true appetite. Instead we are persuaded, or attracted to eat whilst there is still relative satiation, by a variety of external, contextual and social cues. How these factors affect readiness to eat is not well understood. However, it is from eating in this pre-appetite phase of readiness to eat that human 21st century obesity probably arises. Overcoming these external factors is difficult, demanding both conscious wishes and willpower. Certain factors, like alcohol, clearly make the problem worse for some people. Others, like physical activity, probably delay readiness to eat.

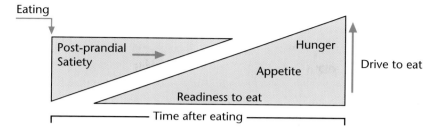

Figure 8 *Proposed hunger–satiety cycle between meals (From Tsofliou et al, unpublished results).*

External and cultural factors, and patterns of weight changes

Medical causes

Lipid, or fat, within adipose tissue, represents the accumulated stored energy (or calories from food) that is not used up immediately after eating. Extra calories from carbohydrate, protein and fat itself are converted into the fat stores in adipose tissue to be used to supply energy (calories) until the next meal, and in the longer term if food supplies dwindle.

Excess body fat storage can only result from a disturbance of energy balance, even when this is a consequence of other medical conditions. Several medical conditions can aggravate weight gain and make obesity more difficult to treat, e.g. untreated hypothyroidism and Cushing's syndrome. Hypothyroidism (underactive thyroid) lowers the metabolic rate to favour a positive energy balance, but seldom causes major weight gain and its correction rarely results in significant weight loss. 'Hypothalamic obesity' can result from a variety of structural problems that affect the appetite or satiety centres in the area of the brain called the hypothalamus; it is extremely rare but can occur after brain injury or in infections such as tuberculosis. Cushing's syndrome involves excessive corticosteroids, either from Cushings disease (the result of a pituitary tumour) or, more commonly, from exogenous steroids used as anti-inflammatory drugs. Steroids can both increase appetite and alter nutrient partitioning to favour fat deposition (centrally) while muscles atrophy, leading to the classical 'lemon-on-matchsticks' body form.

Drugs that cause weight gain

A number of drugs can alter energy balance and promote weight gain, which can be very marked (*Table 4*). The mechanisms may include increase in appetite, or a reduction in energy expenditure. Appetite can be stimulated directly by several drugs, including corticosteroids, antipsychotics needed to treat schizophrenia (particularly atypical antipsychotics) and tricyclic antidepressants, pizotifen for migraine pro-phylaxis, valproate for epilepsy, and progestogens in contraceptive or hormone replacement therapy. Cyproheptadine and megesterol are used to increase appetite in wasted patients and, of course, cause weight gain as an unwanted effect when used for other reasons. Metabolic rate is reduced by beta (β)-adrenoceptor blockers, again causing weight gain. Drugs that stimulate insulin secretion (sulphonylureas) or increase insulin sensitivity (thiazolidine benzedine diones (glitazones)), as well as insulin itself, favour lipogenesis and usually cause weight gain. Many of these drugs are used for conditions which are themselves closely related to weight gain, so drug related weight gain has the potential to aggra-vate the disease being treated.

Table 4 Drugs that may promote weight gain.

Drug	Main condition treated
Insulin	Diabetes
Sulphonylureas	Diabetes
β-adrenergic blockers	Hypertension
Thiazolidene diones (glitazones)	Diabetes
Corticosteroids	Various inflammatory diseases
Cyproheptadine	Allergy, hay fever
Pizotifen	Vasometric headache
Sodium valproate	Epilepsy
Some steroid contraceptives	Contraception
Tricyclic antidepressants	Depression
Atypical anti psychotics	Schizophrenia
Lithium	Bipolar disorder

It should also be remembered that acute weight loss is a frequent feature of many diseases, and suppression of weight gain with chronic illness. When the underlying disease is effectively treated, there will be 'catch up' weight gain.

When drugs known to promote weight gain are prescribed it is important to warn and inform patients. Weight gain is a highly distressing side effect and a common cause of non-compliance. For example, patients are often willing to risk epileptic seizures rather than take sodium valproate and reduce antidiabetic drugs to dangerous levels to avoid weight gain. Nearly all antipsychotic drugs cause weight gain, as much as a mean of 4 kg in 10 weeks (**Table 5**). Weight gain is rated the third worst side effect of atypical antipsychotics (worse than their motor effects), and is the major reason for non-compliance and diabetes development in schizophrenic patients. When any of these drugs causes weight gain, its need and dosage should be re-examined. As in many cases alternative drug classes are available. Whenever these drugs are started, advice on weight control should be given routinely. It is, in principle easier to avoid weight gain by careful choice of low-fat foods and a regular exercise programme, than to try to reverse established weight gain. On medico-legal grounds, the side effects of weight gain needs to be mentioned, that makes preventive management essential.

Table 5 Diabetes associated with significant weight gain in patients taking antipsychotics.

Drug treatment	n	Patients diagnosed with diabetes %
Clozapine	85	15.5
Olanzapine	42	11.0
Haloperidol	60	6.6
Risperidone	58	6.0
Fluphenazine	92	4.5
Other antipsychotics	68	7.3

Appetite, physical activity and food

A large proportion of the calories consumed are used, i.e. oxidized or burnt, unconsciously, as the basal metabolic rate (BMR), to provide energy in the form of adenosine triphosphate (ATP) for breathing and heart beating, and to maintain protein turnover, brain function, etc. Only about one-third of the calories for most individuals is expended on voluntary physical exercise, so the 24-hour energy requirement usually approximates to the BMR $\times$ 1.5. The BMR and the total 24-hour energy expenditure, and thus the number of calories people require, are closely related to body weight. So, if body weight is to remain steady, heavier people generally need more calories than lighter individuals. Overweight people therefore have to eat more calories to avoid weight loss than thinner people: they do not have slow metabolisms. However, metabolic rates, and therefore energy needs, of obesity-prone individuals may be lower before or during the process of weight gain, and be one of the contributory factors to their weight gain. If overweight people lose weight then their metabolic rate is exactly what is predicted by their new weight. As one might expect, overweight people spend less time engaged in physical activity than thinner people; however, they burn more calories, in absolute terms, when they do exercise because they are heavier, and the effort required for movement is greater. The amount of physical activity needed to regulate appetite and prevent weight gain is probably more than most obese people can manage without training.

The decline in physical activity in children, adolescents and adults is a major factor in the increasing rates of obesity, partly because fewer calories are expended, and partly because of a paradoxical elevation of appetite in totally sedentary individuals. Only 8% of UK children now walk to school. Average television watching is 29 hours per week.

For complex psychological and social reasons, overweight people often claim to eat very little, always systematically under-reporting, or under-recording, their food intake. During any period of recording or observation, a shortfall of 20–50% of calories is common, and the under-reporting may be selective for fat. Much scientific confusion has resulted from analyses of dietary intakes of overweight people and attempts to link diet composition with weight change are usually flawed by this under-reporting. This problem is not restricted to the obese. About half of all adults admit to giving misleading information about their food intakes. A surprising number say they tend to over-report food intake, but overweight people, very consistently, under-report it.

The clinician is placed in a difficult position when a significantly over-weight patient claims to eat implausibly few calories. To declare this view risks confrontation and a failure to manage the problem. Similarly, to agree, and accept impossibly low calorie consumption as habitual, may also threaten the therapeutic relationship. Most patients will ultimately agree, after weight loss, that they were not entirely truthful.

Under-reporting is also common in people with a tendency to weight gain, who are struggling with restrained eating, and in elite athletes.

A recent study amongst nurses asked the simple question of whether they would be inclined to under- or over-report their actual food consumption. Amongst nurses with BMI >30 kg/m^2, 51% said that they would intentionally under-report, while 11% said they would over-report; amongst normal-weight nurses (i.e. BMI of 18.5–25 kg/m^2) this pattern was reversed. Across all BMI categories, almost half of ordinary people said they would intentionally give misleading information about their food consumption (*Figure 9*). Evidently, this is a very private domain.

Our appetites are set very carefully for evolutionary reasons, to prevent weight loss at all costs and to promote weight gain whenever there are excess calories available. Appetite is one of the strongest survival forces and without it the human species would have disappeared long ago. It is only when there are excess calories available all the time and people do not have to work physically, that the natural appetite causes problems. The mismatch need only be very small – a 1% error will accumulate 10 000 kcal/year, equivalent to a weight gain of 1–2 kg/year.

Many people are prone to weight gain because they do not notice just how many calories they are consuming, especially from hidden fat in foods, but ultimately their appetite is not switching off at the appropriate point. Several studies have suggested a genetic factor in appetite regulation. For a proportion of patients with underlying psychological disturbances, overeating is a conscious, if secret, way to maintain a social or personal barrier of obesity.

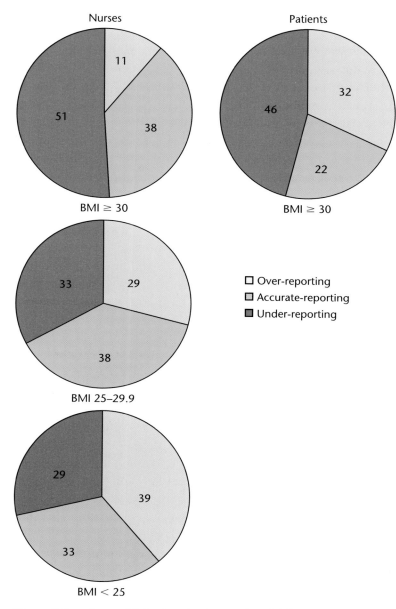

Figure 9 *Prevalence of intentional mis-reporting (%) by BMI category. (Lara et al. unpublished results.)*

Concealing food consumption may reflect a deep-rooted and cross-cultural element in the pursuit of status. Obese people are stigmatized as being of low social status; in many cultures, people (especially women) of high status are portrayed as refined and are seldom seen eating in public, or even to eat normal meal-sized portions if they do. Covert eating has been described in primitive Ethiopian tribes amongst women of high social status, who are not expected to be seen eating. Nursery rhymes, e.g. '. . . a dainty dish to set before a queen' – betray cultural values and concepts of status that reappear in all walks of life.

As may be expected, physical activity also tends to be exaggerated by the obese. For these reasons, it is impossible to establish the level of energy balance of an individual without making physiological measurements. As a general rule, energy intake is best estimated from predicted metabolic rates (based on age, sex and weight) assuming a low level of physical activity.

Genetic predisposition to weight gain

Between individuals, and between communities, there are quite large differences in the predisposition to weight gain, which manifest as differences in prevalences of obesity and overweight. A selection of prevalence data from around the world are shown in *Table 6* and *Figures 10* and *11*. These differences have been examined in studies of migrant communities, and of families and twins, including a large series of twins adopted at birth and reared apart, to conclude that there is a major genetic component behind the predisposition to gain weight. At the same time, it is obviously necessary to have excess calories available if anyone is going to be able to gain weight. A study of adoptees found their BMI (as adults) to be unrelated to the BMI of their adoptive parents but closely related to those of their biological parents (particularly the mothers). Genetic factors thus seem more important than variations in environmental and dietary exposure. This knowledge is vital in order to sympathize with patients' views that their predisposition to weight gain is not entirely their own fault.

Table 6 Obesity prevalence (BMI $\geqslant$ 30 kg/m^2). (Reproduced with permission from Seidell et al[3] and Seidell and Flegal.[4])

Population	Year	Age (Years)	Prevalence of obesity (%) Men	Women
South Africa (Cape Peninsula)				
Blacks	1990	15–64	8	44
Mauritius	1992	25–74	5	15
Rodrigues				
Creoles	1992	25–69	10	31
Tanzania	1986–89	35–64	0.6	3.6
Ghana	1987/88	20+	0.9	0.9
Mali	1991	20+	0.8	0.8
Saudia Arabia	1990–93	15+		
Total			16	24
Urban			18	28
Rural			12	18
Kuwait	1994	18+	32	44
United Arab Emirates	1992	17+	15.8	38
Iran (South)	1993/94	20–74	2.5	7.7
England	1995	16–64	15	16.5
Finland	1991/93	20–75	14	11
Germany	1990	25–69	17	19
Former East Germany	1992	25–69	21	27
West Germany	1991	25–69	16	21
The Netherlands	1995	20–59	8	8
Czech Republic	1988	20–65	16	20
Cyprus	1989/90	35–64	19	24
New Zealand	1989	18–64	10	13
Australia	1989	20–69	9.3	11.1
Japan	1993	20+	1.7	2.7
China	1992	20–45	1.20	1.64
Micronesia				
Nauru	1987	25–69	64.8	70.3
Polynesia				
Western Samoa				
Urban	1991	25–69	58.4	76.8
Rural	1991		41.5	59.2
Melanesia				
Papua New Guinea				
Coastal urban	1991	25–69	36.3	54.3
Coastal rural	1991	25–69	23.9	18.6
Highlands	1991	25–69	4.7	5.3

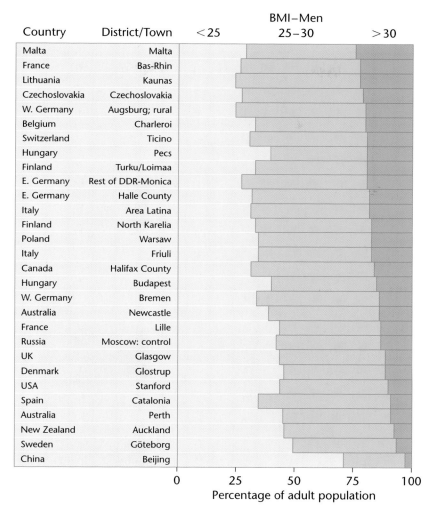

Figure 10 BMI distribution: age standardized proportions of selected categories of men in MONICA populations, age groups 35–64 years over the period 1983–1986. (Adapted from Seidell and Flegal.[4])

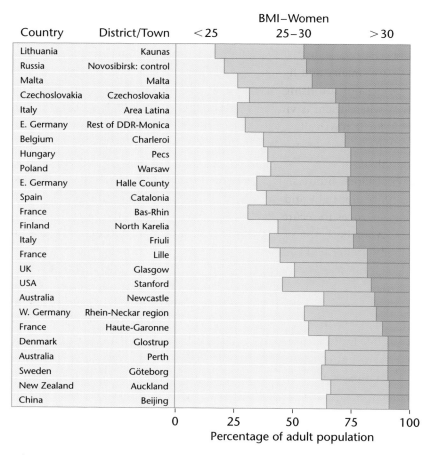

Country	District/Town
Lithuania	Kaunas
Russia	Novosibirsk: control
Malta	Malta
Czechoslovakia	Czechoslovakia
Italy	Area Latina
E. Germany	Rest of DDR-Monica
Belgium	Charleroi
Hungary	Pecs
Poland	Warsaw
E. Germany	Halle County
Spain	Catalonia
France	Bas-Rhin
Finland	North Karelia
Italy	Friuli
France	Lille
UK	Glasgow
USA	Stanford
Australia	Newcastle
W. Germany	Rhein-Neckar region
France	Haute-Garonne
Denmark	Glostrup
Australia	Perth
Sweden	Göteborg
New Zealand	Auckland
China	Beijing

Figure 11 BMI distribution: age standardized proportions of selected categories of women in MONICA populations, age groups 35–64 years over the period 1983–1986. (Adapted from Seidell and Flegal.[4]).

In a successful growing species or society, the biggest single threat to survival is lack of food. Humans have evolved as survivors because of a well-developed mechanism (an appetite that calls for more than is necessary to maintain immediate energy balance) to store calories, when an excess is available, as fat. At c. 7000 kcal/kg, each kilogramme of fat stored can provide for c. 3–4 days of starvation. Most adults, even at a

BMI of 21 kg/m^2, have 7–10 kg of fat stores, which is enough to survive for several weeks with minimal food. Interestingly, both men and women at equivalent BMI have rather similar fat stores, since women, who are smaller and lighter, have a higher proportion of body fat. It is therefore not surprising that most people tend to gain weight in a situation where there is virtually unlimited food and little requirement to work for it physically. It becomes interesting to speculate why a small minority of people appear not to gain weight under the same environmental conditions. It is possible that they perform a social function as long-distance hunters. Our species survives famine by two strategies: firstly, sitting tight and living off fat stores; secondly, running fast and long distances to secure difficult or distant food. In that way, evolution can favour both the obesity-prone and a smaller number of 'constitutionally thin' individuals.

The importance of establishing the existence of genetic factors is that the genes operate by coding proteins, such as hormone receptors for enzymes, and other peptides, such as leptin, which operate as messengers, so there must be metabolic mechanisms responsible for weight problems. In this sense, overweight is a metabolic disease. The metabolic factors may affect energy intake or energy output, i.e. metabolic rate, or (most probably to overcome compensatory mechanisms) both. There is evidence for both types of mechanisms and several proposed factors are listed in *Table 7*. Fat distribution is also partly genetic. For both fatness and fat distribution, the differences between individuals include genetic–environmental interactions such that altering the environment (diet or lifestyle) changes the phenotypic expression.

Specific genes are not yet well established as major causes of simple obesity in humans. In *ob-ob* mice, a single gene defect in leptin production is a cause of obesity. Leptin is a peptide produced in adipose tissue and released, in the well-fed state, to reduce appetite by acting on receptors in the brain. Defects in this system – either in leptin production or in its receptor – cause obesity in congenitally obese rodents. The very recent discovery of the *ob-gene* protein, the appetite-regulator hormone leptin in humans, and its presence in excess in the plasma of overweight subjects (who are evidently resistant to it) has raised another possible

Table 7 Some factors involved in the development of obesity thought to be genetically modulated.

1. Macronutrient related	2. Energy expenditure	3. Hormonal
Adipose tissue lipolysis	Metabolic rate	Insulin sensitivity
Adipose tissue and muscle LPL activity	Thermogenic response to food and other stimuli	Insulin-like growth factors
Muscle composition and oxidative potential	Nutrient partioning	Growth hormone status
Free fatty acid and β-receptor activities in adipose tissue	Propensity for spontaneous physical activity	Leptin action
Capacities for fat and carbohydrate oxidation (respiratory quotient)		
Dietary fat preferences		
Appetite regulation		

endocrine abnormality. Resistance to leptin, allowing excessive eating, could possibly be genetically determined, but the relevance of leptin to simple obesity in humans has not yet been established. Genetic mutations in this system have been found in isolated families with striking parallels to the genetic obesity of the *ob-ob* mouse, but this is very rare. There is some evidence that leptin only regulates appetite in obese people when they undertake physical activity. It is possible that something produced by physical activity allows leptin to enter the brain. Thus when food is available without the need for exercise greater food intake occurs. It is most likely several genetic factors apply in different cases, perhaps acting in concert. It is unlikely (from heritability studies) that a single gene defect is a common cause of being overweight, but it is known to be possible. For example, a deletion on chromosome 15 produces obesity and premature NIDDM in the Prader-Willi syndrome, and several other rare genetic syndromes affecting other chromosomes involve obesity.

Social causes

Prehistory, urbanization and deprivation

In primitive hunter-gatherer societies, most calories were usually provided as carbohydrates rather than as protein, with very small amounts of fat. It is now known that it is dietary fat that is the nutrient most closely linked to weight gain and obesity, while carbohydrate and protein tend to satisfy the appetite better and increase the metabolic rate. It is likely that obesity did not exist at all in the hunter-gatherer era, and BMI in the range of 16–20 kg/m^2 would have been usual. This remains the case for large proportions of the developing world today, with the exception of some individuals who do become overweight and even markedly obese. These overweight individuals are restricted to the most privileged subgroups, particularly those who, for reasons of wealth or caste, do not need to work physically and whose diets probably contain higher than average amounts of fat. Hereditary landowner/farmers, mediaeval churchmen and tax collectors could be viewed as coming into this category, and there are more modern secular equivalents.

Urbanization, with its necessary accompanying industrialization, is the defining feature of an obesity-prone society, and in the twentieth century caused a marked swing away from the association between being overweight and privilege or high social class. In modern Westernized societies, obesity is increasingly a problem of population subgroups characterized by social deprivation *(Figure 12)*. The trend is most marked amongst women, but seems to follow later in men. This trend is particularly worrying, since the same more deprived sectors have elevated health risks from a variety of other associated factors, such as poor housing, smoking, a lack of leisure-time activity facilities and poor diets. The poor diets of the socially deprived has been shaped by poor education and a lack of availability of quality foods, and by a dependence on cheaper foods, which includes a high proportion of high-fat foods. Fat is becoming increasingly a very cheap industrial waste-product of the dairy and meat industries. After maximum profits are made on skimmed milk

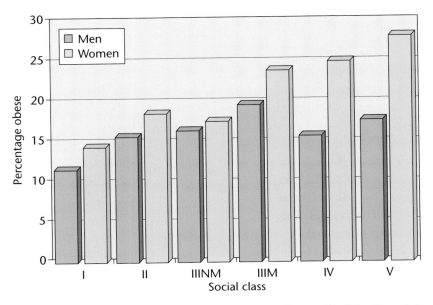

Figure 12 Prevalence of obesity in men and women from each of the six social classes measured by the Health Survey for England 1998. (Source: redrawn with permission from Joint Health Surveys Unit on behalf of the Department of Health (1999). Health Survey for England: Cardiovascular Disease 1998. The Stationary Office: London.[7]

products, fat-trimmed quality cuts, etc., fat can still be marketed to the more deprived sectors, where a cultural value is still placed on dietary fat, in the form of cream, cakes, confectionery and exotic ice creams.

Migrant populations

The cultural influences on attitudes to diet and body shape have been well described in studies of migrant populations. Most international migrant groups have moved from relatively poor and principally rural origins to new urban conditions, and often comprise groups of originally relatively high social position, keen to better themselves. One of the characteristics of migration is weight gain, particularly in women. South Asians who move to the UK, for example, become more overweight than the general British population. Part of this can be attributed to poor social conditions amongst migrants, but the effect is mediated by very low levels of physical activity coupled with a sudden increase in the amount of fat consumed. Cultural attitudes also play a part; e.g. high-fat foods, like meat products and butter, which are prized but scarce in South Asian food culture, suddenly become readily available. South Asians accustomed to spending a very high proportion of their incomes on food migrate to a situation where, in the UK, food is so cheap that only *c.* 12–15% of disposable income is spent on it. There is no cultural value placed on physical activity (either in work or leisure time) in traditional South Asian society, and the body shape considered optimal by women is well above that considered desirable or ideal for health reasons in Western societies. A significant proportion of South Asian women who migrated to Scotland identified a BMI $\geqslant 30$ kg/m^2 as optimal, despite having no experience of such a shape in their own families *(Figure 13)*. They also swung from a low-fat traditional diet to consume an even greater amount of fat than the general Scottish population. However, it is interesting to discover how rapidly some attitudes change: e.g. amongst South Asians in Scotland, the second-generation women born in Scotland had markedly different views about the preferred female shape, coinciding much more closely with the views of the general population, and they also modified their eating habits to reduce fat consumption towards that of the general population.

Epidemiology

A recent WHO consultation on obesity has collected a large number of surveys on prevalence of overweight and BMI, a selection of which are shown in *Figures 10* and *11*. These studies may not all be completely representative of the countries concerned, but were all conducted using good quality methods, so these data do give a good indication of the variations between countries. In developed countries, the proportion of adults with a BMI of 25–30 kg/m^2 is the biggest sector. This proportion is reasonably constant in size between countries and represents a rather larger proportion in men than in women. The proportion of adults with

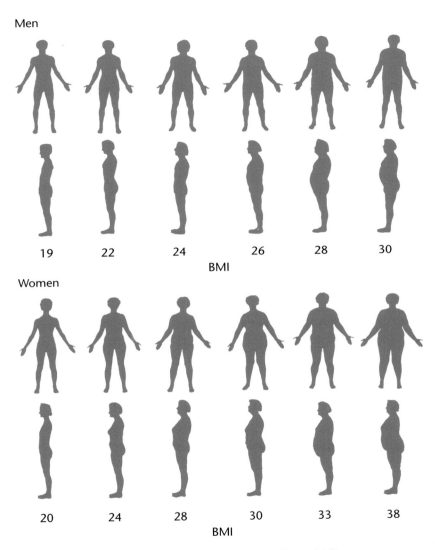

Figure 13 *Photographic silhouettes of adults of different BMI.*

BMI > 30 kg/m² is more variable, with a wider range extending to much greater prevalences amongst women. Thus, across much of the world, variations in BMI profiles occur through reciprocal differences amongst the proportions who are obese and those who are thin or normal. This global pattern tends to suggest that our genes are usually directed towards a BMI of 25–30 kg/m² (i.e. overweight) and this explains how obesity becomes a problem as soon as undernourishment has been abolished.

The highest levels of obesity are now seen in Polynesian communities, up to 70% with BMI > 40 kg/m². Other small-island communities and places like Kuwait, which produce no natural food, follow closely behind. The former Eastern block countries exhibit the highest rates of obesity in Europe, but isolated Western regions in Malta, Germany and Italy also show high prevalences. The lowest rates of obesity are in developing countries, and in Japan, China, Australia and New Zealand. The highly-educated Swedish city of Göteborg has a notably low prevalence of obesity. The USA population, which is popularly portrayed as being generally obese, clearly has a large unseen thin sector, so the average is not particularly high on a world scale. *Table 6* shows data on recent trends in obesity prevalence. Virtually all are increasing rapidly, albeit from different starting points between countries.

chapter 4

The burden of ill health from obesity

The overall burden of ill health that results from overweight and obesity reflects both their high prevalences and also the astonishing range of specific health problems that they cause or aggravate. Problems increase with age. Virtually all people with a BMI > 30 kg/m^2 (waist > 88 cm in women or > 102 cm in men) develop some physical symptoms by about the age of 40, as well as frequent depression, and the majority require medical attention or drug therapy for secondary conditions by the age of 50 or 60. Half of all men with a waist > 94 cm or women with a waist > 80 cm have at least one major risk factor for coronary heart disease (CHD) and strokes. Additionally, there is the elevated likelihood of overweight people developing other life-threatening diseases, including sleep apnoea, cellulitis, thrombosis and a range of major cancers.

These different components of the total burden of ill health attributable to weight gain have a very real impact on the individual and on health services, and there is a major social and societal cost that is often difficult to measure, and seldom fully appreciated by those who do not recognize the full complexity of the disease.

Direct symptoms from overweight and obesity

Physical symptoms of obesity
When overweight people visit a doctor it is not usually through worry

about increased risks for fatal diseases but rather because of symptoms they are experiencing. These may be symptomatic aggravations of other conditions, symptoms of secondary complications of obesity or symptoms of overweight itself.

The commonest symptoms of overweight *per se* are *shortness of breath* on minor exertion, such as walking up stairs or hills, *difficulty in sleeping, low back pain, hip and knee pain, tiredness* and *depression.* Some symptoms are sensitive or embarrassing, and might be missed without careful history taking: *stress incontinence* may be present in > 61% of overweight patients; *menstrual disturbances,* including menorrhagia and oligomenorrhoea, and *infertility* are common; an excess of *hirsute* patients are overweight; *sweating* is increased through an elevated metabolic rate and contributes to skin problems, including oppositional intertrigo. Above a BMI 40 kg/m² it is often difficult to maintain normal cleanliness.

The range of symptoms that can be directly attributed to overweight extends across most major medical specialty areas. Most are not symptoms specific to overweight and other common diseases may be mimicked. Many of the symptoms are related both to the degree of overweight and to age, and are often suppressed in medical consultation because of their insidious development. It is relatively uncommon for patients to volunteer symptoms of obesity under about the age of 40; when they do, either obesity is extreme or another underlying disease is likely to be present. It is also relatively uncommon for patients to recognize direct symptoms, apart from limited mobility and exercise capacity, while the BMI is < 30 kg/m². On direct questioning, symptoms are often much more common than initially revealed and they contribute significantly to an impairment of quality of life. Very broadly, the medical hazards of obesity can be classified as resulting from *mechanical, metabolic* or *mental effects,* although a number of complications involve combinations of these effects *(Table 8).*

Low back pain and joint pain

Low back and joint pains probably present the largest component of the burden of obesity on health services. This is mainly a mechanical problem – pain resulting from accelerated joint damage as well as aggravated

Table 8 Medical consequences of overweight and obesity.

Physical symptoms	Metabolic problems	Anaesthetic/surgical	Endocrine problems	Social problems	Psychological problems
Tiredness	Hypertension	Sleep apnoea	Hirsutism	Isolation	Low self-esteem
Breathlessness	NIDDM	Chest infections	Oligomenorrhea/infertility	Agoraphobia	Self-deception
Varicose veins	Hepatic steatosis	Wound dehiscence	Metromenorrhagia	Unemployment	Cognitive disturbance
Back pain	Hyperlipidaemia	Hernia	Oestrogen-dependent	Family/marital stress	Distorted body image
Oedema/cellulitis	Hypercoagulation	Venous thrombosis	cancers, i.e. breast,	Discrimination	Depression
Sweating/intertrigo	Ischaemic heart		uterus, prostate		
Stress incontinence	disease and stroke				

symptoms. There is, however, an ill-understood metabolic effect as well, such that osteoarthritis of the hands is more frequent in the overweight. A link with gout (also more common in the obese) has been suggested. Symptoms of low back pain and intervertebral disc herniation affect *c.* 50% of all adults at some stage every year, and there is a remarkable association between the degree of overweight, reflected either by BMI or waist circumference measurements, both in terms of the prevalence of symptoms and in terms of the consequences for employment *(Table 9)*.

Indigestion

Indigestion has an increased frequency in the overweight, related to their higher likelihood of hiatus hernia, a mechanical effect of an increased mass of abdominal fat, rather than an effect on oesophageal reflux *per se*. A very common cause of peptic ulcer and indigestion generally is *Helicobacter pylori* infection of the stomach. *H. pylori* infection rates and peptic ulceration are not increased amongst the obese, indeed, *H. pylori* is, if anything, more associated with undernourishment on a global basis.

Table 9 Proportions of Dutch adults whose daily lives were affected due to low back pain the past 12 months (n = 2467 men, 3448 women) in different categories of body mass index (BMI), adjusted for age, smoking and education. (From Han et al.[8])

	Men BMI (kg/m²)			Women BMI (kg/m²)		
	<25	25–30	≥30	<25	25–30	≥30
Proportions (%)†	(42.1)	(46.2)	(11.7)	(56.0)	(31.9)	(12.2)
Daily business hindered	28.2	27.4	34.9*	25.3	30.2**	32.3**
Absence from work	25.4	23.0	27.6	18.8	23.2*	28.4**
Medication consultation	39.3	40.9	40.5	39.6	44.7**	45.7**
Job redundancy	11.2	12.2	15.2	8.2	9.2	10.9

*Difference from Body mass index < 25 kg/m²: ** p < 0.01; *p < 0.05*
†Proportions of subjects in each BMI category

Urinary incontinence

In women, urinary incontinence is probably mainly mechanical. Incontinence starts usually as stress, or occasionally as urge, incontinence, with BMI > 30 kg/m²; it is more frequent in older patients. It is often an undisclosed symptom, but is a major source of unhappiness and embarrassment and is surprisingly common. One American study found incontinence in 61% of women with a mean BMI of 33.1 kg/m².[9] Weight loss reduced then to 10%.

Menstrual disturbances

A range of menstrual disturbances are more frequent in overweight than in normal weight women. These are mediated by elevated leptin, which contributes importantly to early menarche, and elevated free androgens and/or oestrogens, resulting from low sex-hormone-binding globulins and increased aromatase activity in adipose tissue. Infertility is more common and metromenorrhagia can be problematic. Infertility treatment is often unsuccessful in the obese.

Breathlessness

Breathlessness is a very common and characteristic complaint in the overweight. It may indicate an aggravation from excess weight of underlying respiratory disease, but more often it constitutes a direct symptom of overweight *per se* in people with no lung disease. It is partly mechanical – very overweight people find it harder to breathe – and partly metabolic – an elevated metabolic rate means that they need more oxygen and have to dispose of more CO_2, just as is the case for anybody carrying a heavy load. The effects of overweight and smoking are additive *(Figure 14)*. Respiratory infections, particularly postoperatively, are also more common in the overweight.

Major medical hazards of obesity

Sleep apnoea syndrome and Pickwickian syndrome

Sleep apnoea is related to the breathlessness of obesity, and is a potentially fatal and frequently unrecognized condition. It is characterized by

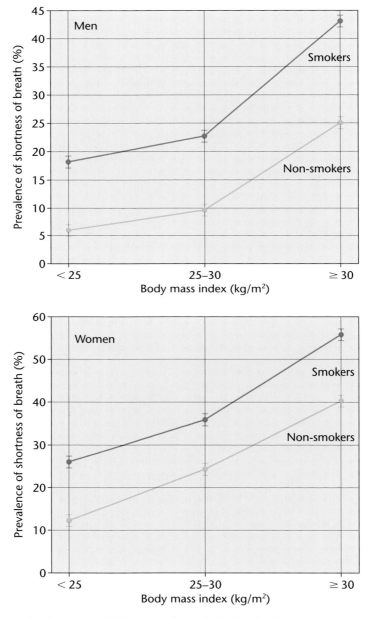

Figure 14 *Prevalence of shortness of breath in Dutch adults.*

periods of apnoea during sleep, which are often first recognized by a partner. The patient may report waking gasping for breath and may be misdiagnosed as having pulmonary oedema. Warning signs include snoring and waking up feeling unrefreshed (because of poor sleeping or hypoxia during sleep). Pickwickian syndrome – characterized by obese patients falling asleep inappropriately (even when driving) – is a well-described consequence. Road traffic accidents are more common in the overweight – a consequence of overweight drivers falling asleep more often. People prone to Pickwickian syndrome may be those with altered CO_2 drive to respiration.

There are several components to the pathophysiology of sleep apnoea syndrome. It is probably necessary to have both a relatively insensitive respiratory centre (alcohol may aggravate this) and also a mechanical obstruction to respiration, such as palatal dysfunction, massive obesity or marked central fat distribution. Adipose tissue in the neck is increased when there is a central fat distribution (both intraabdominal and neck fat are derived from the brown adipose tissue of infancy). Sleep apnoea syndrome can be mimicked by applying elastic bands around the chest. Even in healthy people there is normally some reduction in arterial oxygen tension overnight: in the worst cases of sleep apnoea syndrome this is exaggerated and death may occur through hypoxic cardiac arrhythmias. Hypoxic convulsions may occur during sleep apnoea and patients tend to respond poorly to anticonvulsants.

Oedema of the legs

Oedema of the legs may develop in obesity without any underlying cardiac or renal failure, or sodium retention, and it responds poorly to diuretic therapy. Venous stasis is more common in the overweight, partly through lower mobility and partly through venous occlusion from fat at the inguinal canal. Cyclical oedema in women is poorly understood but is clearly related to obesity; it does not respond well to diuretics but is controlled by weight loss.

Cellulitis

Cellulitis is a common and serious complication in the very overweight, which complicates and compounds the problem of oedema, setting up a vicious cycle through damage to the lymphatic system. Cellulitis tends to respond more slowly to antibiotics in seriously obese patients. It is an important cause of major morbidity and death in severely obese patients.

Anaesthetic and surgical hazards

Anaesthesia and surgery present a familiar catalogue of increased risk to the overweight, including an increased likelihood of chest infections, wound infections, dehiscence, herniation, postoperative back pain and thromboembolism. These risks provide a frequent reason for denying elective surgery to obese individuals, often with unrealistic demands for weight loss. There are clearly some surgical operations whose success would be highly unlikely in seriously overweight patients, e.g. a knee replacement for arthritis. In others, such as thoracotomy or laparotomy, the increased hazards may demand the availability of ventilatory intensive care or high-dependency postoperative support. Guidelines for day surgery usually include an upper limit of a BMI of 30 kg/m^2, above which more prolonged admission is required because of the increased perioperative risks.

Venous thrombosis

Venous thrombosis is increased in the overweight, reflecting their altered metabolic aspects, e.g. elevated haemostatic factors (such as fibrinogen and factor VII) and reduced thrombolytic factors (such as increased plasminogen activator inhibitor).

Thrombosis risk is also elevated by venous stasis and oedema as a mechanical effect of obesity.

Cardiovascular diseases (heart disease and stroke)

Cardiovascular diseases are clearly increased in the overweight and represent the main reasons for increased mortality. Although the relative risks are fairly small and very large studies have been required to prove the links, because of the enormous incidences of these diseases the impact of overweight is important in leading to vast numbers of extra heart attacks and strokes each year. Obesity has effects by aggravating several of the causal risk factors, including high blood pressure and high blood cholesterol, resulting in atheroma formation. It aggravates the tendency to thrombosis, by elevating coagulation factor VII, and it is the main preventable cause of NIDDM, which aggravates both atheroma in large vessels and thrombosis risk.

The presence of obesity has a very significant effect, approximately doubling cardiovascular risk at BMI > 30 kg/m^2 when other risk factors are absent, but in the presence of other major risk factors this influence is enormously exaggerated *(Figure 15)*. Long-term follow-up studies have shown that weight gain in childhood and adolescence is important, but the greatest hazards come from weight gain in adult life.

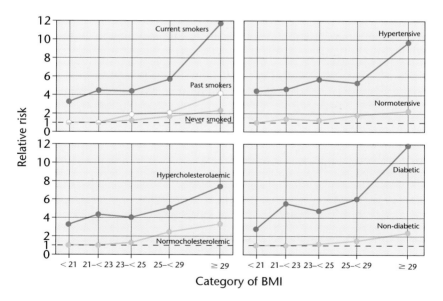

Figure 15 *Relative risks of nonfatal myocardial infarction and fatal coronary heart disease (combined), in middle-aged women according to BMI and coronary risk factor status, after adjustment for age and smoking. The risks are significantly elevated in those without the risk factor, and greatly compounded in those with the risk factor. (Reproduced with permission from Manson et al.[10])*

Diabetes and impaired glucose tolerance

The influence of being overweight on diabetes is truly spectacular. It usually develops before BMI 30 kg/m² is reached – at an average BMI of 29 in the UK. The likelihood of NIDDM at BMI >25 kg/m² is increased eight-fold, and at BMI >30 kg/m² 40-fold, compared with that at a BMI of 22 kg/m² *(Figure 16)*. Longitudinal studies show that diabetes in later life is predicted from a patient being overweight as a teenager, but most of the risk is from weight gain as an adult. From large studies by Willett and colleagues[12] in Boston, USA, it is estimated that well over half of all diabetes would be abolished if weight gain in adults could be prevented. Even within the acceptable range of BMI, weight loss for people with a BMI in the range of 23–25 kg/m² reduces the incidence of NIDDM.

The major clinical problem of type 2 diabetes is accelerated heart disease, but this is already present before the diagnostic criteria for

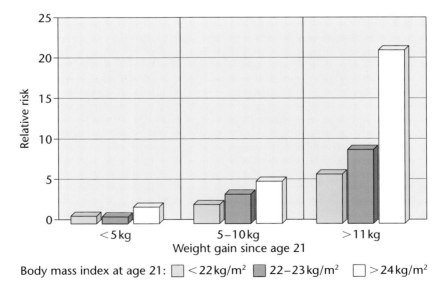

Figure 16 The relative risk of developing diabetes in men increases within each tertile of weight gain and within each category of BMI at age 21. (Adapted from Chan et al.[11])

diabetes are reached, i.e. with impaired glucose tolerance. The greatest burden of disease is in people with BMI in, or just above, the normal range.

Cancers

Overweight is now increasingly being recognized as a major preventable cause of a range of major cancers, including colon, breast, endometrial and prostate. It is estimated that 35% of all cancers, including several very major cancers that lead to 70% of all cancer deaths, have nutritional links, and overweight is an important factor. All these cancers have multifactorial aetiologies and obesity can play several roles. In colonic cancer there is an interaction between dietary fat and obesity, and associations with physical inactivity have also been reported. The other major obesity-related cancers (breast, uterus, ovary and prostate) are under some endocrine regulation that is altered in the overweight. In adipose tissue there is an enzyme, aromatase, that converts adrenal steroids into androgens in women, and androgens to oestrogenic metabolites in men. Expanded adipose tissue leads to excess expression of aromatase and a trophic effect on these cancers is mediated by the sex hormone metabolites. Sex-hormone-binding globulins are reduced in the obese, so circulating free oestrogens are particularly elevated.

Mortality and life expectancy

Mortality risks, overall, are increased in overweight people *(Figure 2)*. Survival of young people starts to decline as soon as their weight is increased above normal for their height. This occurs when the BMI is >25 kg/m^2, or when the waist circumference exceeds 80 cm (32 in) for a woman or 94 cm (37 in) for a man. The increased mortality is mainly a result of known associations with conditions such as diabetes, heart disease and stroke, although additional cancers are also important. For older people, the link between obesity and reduced survival is not so strong. The main adverse consequences of overweight in older people are the symptoms associated with being overweight and not the increased risks to life expectancy.

The mortality links between overweight and premature death have been borne out in several very large longitudinal studies. The Framingham Study[13] identified overweight as being similar in importance to smoking in predicting premature death. Most of the effect is through accelerated cardiovascular disease. High waist circumference was a slightly more powerful predictor of death than BMI (at least in men), presumably because it incorporates risks associated with central fat distribution as well as just fatness. In broad terms, having a BMI >30 kg/m^2, or a waist circumference of >102 cm (40 in) in men or >88 cm (35 in) in women, means having at least double the mortality risk of people of a normal weight, i.e. a BMI of 18.5–25 kg/m^2.

Mental problems of overweight and obesity: quality of life

For somebody who is overweight, the qualify of life is obviously impaired by the symptoms outlined above, but it is also influenced by the way in which overweight people are treated by others, and by a lack of self-esteem that results from being unable to do things as quickly or as easily as other people. This, in turn, leads to discrimination, reduced prospects and social isolation. Low self-esteem has been reported to result from even very minor cases of relative overweight in 11-year-old children: it affects school performance and social development, and the effects often remain for life.

The psychological effects of being overweight are profound and very complicated. For some people, overeating is an almost conscious reaction to other psychological stresses, e.g. an unhappy marriage, psychological trauma in childhood or stress at work, but this group is a minority. Boredom can produce internal cues that the individual interprets as hunger but which might in fact be satisfied by physical activity. Continued overeating by the overweight is partly hyperphagia as a physiological response to continuous discrimination in every walk of life. A very large Swedish study measured quality of life, using a variety of standard measures, and found that obesity (BMI >30 kg/m^2) led to a worse quality of life, with more stress and anxiety, than having rheumatoid arthritis, tetraplegia or a disseminated malignancy.[14] An American study found that the physical pain – throughout the body – experienced by obese people was similar to that of migraine sufferers.[15] Obesity is very distressing: a jolly smiling fat man or woman is usually only smiling for the camera.

Tiredness is a very common symptom in the overweight. General factors contribute, including the effort of moving excess weight, the chronically high metabolic rate, and poor sleeping associated with snoring and the sleep apnoea syndrome. Boredom in the overweight is often labelled as depression. Depression itself does occur commonly as a self-reported problem in the overweight, but the aetiological links are often disputed. It seems that obesity does not usually occur as a consequence of pre-existing depression, but rather that the tiredness, poor quality of life, symptoms and social discrimination experienced by overweight people conspire to generate chronic unhappiness and low self-esteem. Although the term 'depression' is often used by both patients and doctors, it is unlike the 'endogenous depression' recognized by psychiatrists, in several ways. With endogenous depression weight loss is usual, not weight gain. Obese patients who complain of depression seldom score highly on diagnostic criteria and/or by psychiatrists, and they are seldom helped by anti-depressant medications.

chapter 5

Clinical benefits of weight loss

Many symptoms that result from immediate mechanical and metabolic consequences of obesity respond rapidly to weight loss *(Table 8)*. For some, a complete cure is possible with major weight loss, but symptoms are often banished and risk factors corrected by losses of 5–10 kg.

It is important to consider the amount of weight loss needed to bring benefit, and to distinguish between the effects of active weight loss, i.e. acute negative energy balance, usually in the context of frequent professional contact, and the effects of having lost weight and then maintaining that new stable level. Over prolonged periods of observation, the subsequent effects of age and weight regain need to be considered.

Reducing symptoms

For most people with weight problems, what really matters is feeling better, generally fitter and sharper, and having fewer of the symptoms resulting from being overweight. These are therefore the most important criteria on which to judge a weight-management programme or treatment. From several large analyses, it is now recognized that it is not necessary to lose all excess weight or to achieve a normal-weight target in order to improve symptoms. Amongst the first symptoms to improve with weight loss are sweating, breathlessness, tiredness and diabetic symptoms – often even before the weight loss is detectable. Angina, which often occurs without demonstrable coronary disease in the obese, improves with only 5% weight loss. Menstrual disturbances, including menorrhagia, oligomenorrhoea and infertility, all improve with a weight loss of 7 kg (15 lb), and within 2 months. Those with arthritis or back pain will find improvement with a similar loss. Stress incontinence can be reduced from *c*. 60 to 10% in women with a BMI of 33 kg/m². More sustained weight loss is necessary to correct NIDDM, hirsutism and sleep apnoea completely, but clinically important and symptomatic improvements occur after a weight loss of 5–10 kg *(Table 10)*. It must, however, be explained to patients that the process of weight loss, i.e. being in acute negative energy balance, is uncomfortable and commonly causes tiredness or irritability.

Table 10 Symptomatic improvment with weight loss.

Symptoms of obesity usually relieved by a weight loss of 5–10 kg

Tiredness
Back pain
Joint pain: hips and knees
Angina
Sweating
Breathlessness
Snoring
Menstrual symptoms (menorrhagia, amenorrhoea)
Infertility
Stress incontinence
Polydipsia/polyuria with NIDDM

Symptoms that may require a weight loss > 5–10 kg.

Sleep apnoea
Leg oedema/cellulitis
Hirsutism

Quality of life and self-esteem

The depressive symptoms so common in the overweight are partly a consequence of having failed (and been treated as a failure by others) in attempts to control a weight problem. Perhaps the most rewarding end product for people who successfully lose some weight, and then maintain a lower weight, is the boost in morale and self-esteem. This, coupled with the improvement in symptoms and the knowledge that health risks have been reduced, can contribute to a marked improvement in overall quality of life, including improved social life. It is important to recognize how hard it is for an obese patient to lose 5–10% of their weight and it should be made clear that this is to be regarded as a major success, to be rewarded and maintained. Continued professional contact and support, and encouragement from friends and families all contribute to these improvements.

Future health: reducing risk factors and disease

The major metabolic risk factors in people with diabetes – blood lipids, blood pressure and blood glucose – are all affected by an acute energy balance, and are also predictably improved in relation to the amount of weight lost. Risk factors improve most in people at highest risk, i.e. those with the highest risk factors, or those who can be identified as having the most marked central fat distribution. Thus, people with the biggest waist circumferences derive the greatest benefit from weight loss, and this provides a good reason to use the waist circumference measurement in screening and health promotion.

It is important to note that the most rapid and marked improvements in cardiovascular risk factors occurs during acute energy restriction, i.e. in the acute phase of slimming, and often before detectable weight loss. The risk factors then tend to settle to a new intermediate level with sustained weight loss. The one exception to this is high-density lipoprotein (HDL), which falls acutely during active energy restriction and then rises once weight has stabilized. Recognizing the acute changes in total and low-density lipoprotein (LDL) cholesterol helps to explain why quite dramatic improvements are claimed in short-term studies, where active weight loss is continuing at the time of follow-up measurement. Studies lasting > 3–4 months usually produce more modest improvements, probably because weight has actually stabilized at the time of the final measurements. The reduction in blood pressure is related partly to loss of weight and partly to a reduction in salt intake during acute energy restriction, which occurs in healthier diets. Systolic, diastolic and mean arterial pressures all fall by a similar proportion.

A weight loss of 5–10 kg (*c.* 15 lb) brings very definite health benefits; in fact, most benefits that are potentially achievable by weight loss are achieved with the first 5–10 kg loss. A significant (> 10%) improvement in at least one major cardiovascular risk factor (high blood pressure, high cholesterol, low HDL) has been shown in 80% of overweight patients who lose 5–10 kg *(Table 11)*.

Table 11 Clinical benefits of weight loss.

Cardiovascular risk-factor improvement with sustained weight loss.

	Change per kg loss (%)	Change with 5–10 kg loss (%)
Total cholesterol	−1	−5
LDL cholesterol	−2	−5
HDL cholesterol	+1 to +2	+10 to +15
Triglycerides	−2 to −5	−10 to −25
Blood pressure	−1 to −2	−5 to −10
Coagulation factor VII	−1	−5 to −10
Red-cell aggregation	−2	−10 to −15

Other long-term benefits from weight loss

Better wound healing	Lower mortality
Fewer chest infections	Reduced oedema
Less destructive osteoarthritis	Greater mobility
Less prone to NIDDM	Reduced angina
Less thromboembolism	

Most of the risk factors for cardiovascular disease are aggravated by weight gain, improve with weight loss, but also deteriorate with age. Blood pressure will fall with weight loss, but tends to climb again over a period of years, even with weight maintenance. Without any interventions blood pressure would have been even higher.

Several very large studies have recently reported the enormous reduction in incidence of type 2 diabetes which results from weight management. For overweight people with impaired glucose, a diet tolerance and lifestyle programme (involving regular walking) which reduces body weight by about 5 kg reduces new cases of diabetes by almost 60% over 4 years.[16,17] Addition of orlistat reduces weight a further 2–3 kg, and adds a further 30–40% reduction in new diabetes. Gastric surgery, with colossal weight loss, has even greater effect,[18] but these diet and exercise programmes should be acceptable and accessible to large numbers of people. The cost savings from prevention of diabetes are colossal, as well as reductions in disabilities.

Increasing life expectancy

How weight loss modifies survival of life expectancy has been a topic of debate and some confusion in the past. In part, this is because it was not possible in epidemiological studies that enquire about previous weight change to distinguish between the effects of intentional weight loss and those losses as a result of illness. However, large American follow-up studies have shown that while unintentional weight loss is clearly associated with illness and premature death, intentional weight loss leads mainly to improved health and reduced mortality in the general population. The benefits are greatest in people with pre-existing obesity-related conditions. In patients with NIDDM, weight loss under advice is clearly linked to increased survival *(Figure 17)*. Each 1 kg of weight lost translates to 3–4 months increased life expectancy for the average diabetic patient who presents with a BMI >25 kg/m^2. A 10 kg loss restores life expectancy to non-diabetic levels.

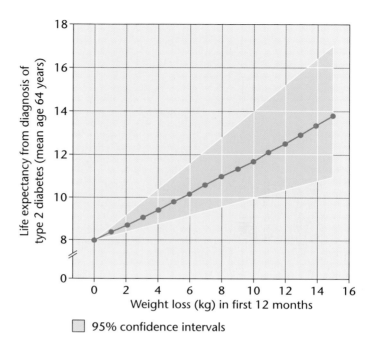

Figure 17 Weight loss in the first year of treatment improves the prognosis of overweight (BMI > 25 kg/m²) patients with NIDDM with a median age of 64 at diagnosis, followed until death. (Reproduced with permission from Lean et al.[19])

The benefits of intentional weight loss on mortality in women are summarized in *Figure 18*. Unintentional weight loss, in the same study, increased mortality, but the value of intentional weight loss is very striking, especially for patients with obesity-related diseases. For men this major benefit again lay amongst those with diabetes.

This recent research has reduced concern about the supposed mortality risks of yo-yo dieting, however, the evidence is entirely based on reported weight change for any reason, including illness. People in large population surveys who report previous swings in weight have more heart disease and cancers, so weight cycling of this kind is often associated with existing disease, either an unintended consequence or perhaps a deliberate attempt to lose weight because of health

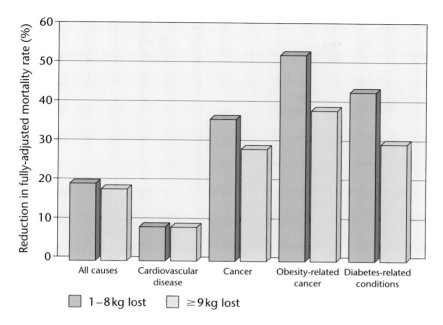

Figure 18 *Intentional weight loss results in significantly reduced mortality rates for women with obesity-related health problems. (Reproduced with permission from Williamson et al.[20])*

problems. Many people with weight problems do habitually diet to lose weight and then regain it, repeating this cycle many times during adult life. Yo-yo dieting of this kind may or may not result in a lower weight than would have developed without dieting, and may be stressful. It has been found that it can reduce bone mineral mass, so perhaps contributing to osteoporosis later on, but there is no direct evidence about long-term health from healthy people who go through deliberate dieting of this kind. Advice to avoid weight cycling is appropriate and should form part of a major emphasis on avoidance of weight gain or regain after loss.

Benefits from weight loss may reflect independent effects from different components of a weight-loss programme. For example, diet composition has independent effects on lipids, blood pressure and thrombotic tendency, and these effects add long-term benefit, even when relatively little weight loss is achieved. Physical activity reduces resting blood pressure, increased HDL cholesterol and reduces triglyceride independently of any weight loss. It reduces the likelihood of developing NIDDM and improves all indices of diabetic control (glycaemic and lipid) in people with diabetes. It increases life expectancy in patients with insulin dependent diabetes mellitus (IDDM) and may be expected to have a similar effect in NIDDM.

chapter 6

Clinical guidelines for weight management

Obesity and a degree of overweight that produce symptoms and secondary complications develop in about a half of all adults. The health problems that develop can manifest in patients who come under the management of a complete range of medical and surgical sub-specialties. Obesity and weight management have not conventionally been taught as a specialty subject in medical schools, and only very recently have professional organizations begun to bring clinicians interested in weight management together. It is now becoming clear, giving the immense personal, social and health care costs of overweight and obesity, that more effective management is required. Weight gain represents the consequence of many interacting processes and, as such, obesity is a disease with a multifactorial aetiology. This being the case, there will always be different approaches to its management that are more or less effective to different individuals. In this setting, the need to provide guidance for clinicians in weight management has begun to emerge as a priority issue.

Clinical guidelines have been viewed with suspicion by all parties (i.e. doctors, patients or patient organizations and commercial organizations with an interest). The legal status of guidelines comes into question when things go wrong or when trust is lost in a therapeutic relationship.

The status of clinical guidelines depends very much on the context, the terms used and the status of the issuing body. In principle, guidelines are written to make scientific evidence available and to allow its translation into practical management by clinicians. There are two rather different situations in which guidelines are required or desirable. The first is the situation where a given treatment is clearly superior to alternative forms of management and where this treatment should be given to every patient. An extreme example might be the treatment with an antibiotic (usually penicillin) for meningococcal septicaemia. In this situation, the potential need for guidelines would relate to the threshold criteria for diagnosis upon which treatment should be started. Even in the absence of formal guidelines, failure to observe conventionally-accepted diagnostic criteria would probably be regarded as evidence of neglect or malpractice. For conditions such as this example, formal clinical guidelines may not, in fact, be required.

A second situation under which clinical guidelines may be sought is when more than one potential treatment exists for a condition and for which none is ideal. This is particularly evident where personality and lifestyle form part of the management. In this setting, the scientific evidence is often difficult to evaluate and its application to an individual case by an individual clinician may require some flexibility.

Clinical guidelines usually carry some implications for resource management. Very often, guidelines are restricted to the treatment of a diagnosis and may need to be interpreted in the context of the whole human being. For these reasons, the guidelines produced by a disease-specific organization, e.g. guidelines for the management of hyperlipidaemia produced by a hyperlipidaemia association or guidelines for the management of diabetes produced by a diabetes association, are likely to have different emphases from guidelines produced either by a central medical organization, e.g. in the UK, the Department of Health, Health Service Executive or one of the Royal Colleges. These emphases will again be modified in guidelines produced by a care-provider organization such as a hospital, or by primary care organizations. The reason for local guidelines is usually on grounds of resource limitations and has led to iniquitous postcode prescribing. To try to avoid this, national guidelines are now being produced in UK, attempting to weigh up clinical efficacy, hazards and cost-effectiveness, by NICE (National Institute for Clinical Excellence) and the Health Technology Board for Scotland.

One problem with such a system is that a wide range of skills and an understanding of complex diseases are required.

In recent years, clinical guidelines for obesity and weight management have been published by several organizations in different countries. In the USA and Germany, recommendations have been made by organizations representing obesity management. The American recommendations, published by the Institute of Medicine (1995), have important input from patient organizations and were followed by the National Institutes of Health evidence-based guidelines for clinical practice.[21] In the UK, clinical guidelines have been produced by a working party from the Royal Colleges based in Scotland.[22]

The status of the Scottish Intercollegiate Guidelines Network (SIGN) guidelines on weight management is set out clearly. They are based on scientific evidence using a grading system that originates from the US Agency of Health Care Policy and Research *(Table 12)*. The targets of these guidelines are practising doctors, but already they have had an impact on policy-makers and paramedical health professions, and they have been reported in the general press. Initially, new guidelines do not immediately lead to changes in practice, but improved care is likely when patients start to demand it.

Table 12 lists the type of evidence required for different grades of recommendation. It is interesting to observe that the criteria required for Grade A research under this system can seldom be met in studies that look at the benefits of weight reduction. This is because it is impossible to provide a placebo, since part of the treatment is dietary and lifestyle modification, and the criteria were originally conceived for judging drug treatment. A second reason for difficulty in applying conventional evidence criteria is that weight loss cannot be considered a point intervention and it is never a fixed-dose treatment. Thus, weight loss varies in extent between individuals and the duration of treatment is a critical part of the evaluation. These points are not immediately apparent to analysts unfamiliar with the field. At least one prominently published meta-analysis of weight loss in diabetic patients has produced rather confused conclusions because of a failure to appreciate these points.

Table 12 Grading system for recommendations adopted for the SIGN guidelines. (Reproduced with permission of SIGN.[22])

Grade	Recommendation
A	**Required:** At least one radomized controlled trial as part of the body of literature of overall good quality and consistency addressing specific recommendation
B	**Required:** Availability of well-conducted clinical studies but no randomized clinical trials on the topic of recommendation
C	**Required:** Evidence obtained from expert committee reports or opinions and/or clinical experiences of respected authorities. Indicates absence of directly applicable clinical studies of good quality

The purpose of the guidelines on obesity produced by the SIGN Working Party for the Royal Colleges in Scotland was the first set of evidence-based obesity management guidelines in 1996. They aimed to provide a blueprint that would lead to the development of local practices after local resource evaluation. It was planned that a review of the guidelines should be produced every 2 years, taking new evidence into account, but the revision was abandoned. The weight-management scheme produced in the pilot SIGN guidelines is specifically headed as being for guidance only, to provide a logical management process to evaluate and modify the need for a centre in the country. Because a management scheme of this type has not previously been proposed or tested, the entire scheme is considered to represent Grade C evidence as a recommendation from an expert committee.

The weight-management scheme *(Figure 19)* presents an idealized model aimed at management and control of one of the world's leading causes of disease and disability, based at the level of primary care. Underlying this emphasis is the view that the principle mode of management is through lifestyle factors and that one of the most insistent themes running through the literature is that regular professional contact gives the strongest predictor for success. It is therefore

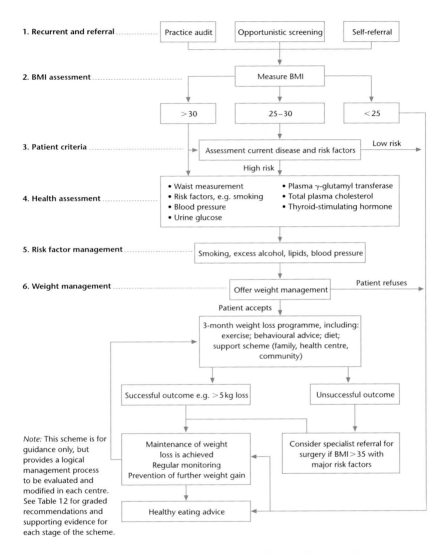

1. Recurrent and referral .... | Practice audit | Opportunistic screening | Self-referral |

2. BMI assessment .... Measure BMI

> 30 | 25–30 | < 25

3. Patient criteria .... Assessment current disease and risk factors — Low risk

High risk

4. Health assessment ....
- Waist measurement
- Risk factors, e.g. smoking
- Blood pressure
- Urine glucose
- Plasma γ-glutamyl transferase
- Total plasma cholesterol
- Thyroid-stimulating hormone

5. Risk factor management .... Smoking, excess alcohol, lipids, blood pressure

6. Weight management .... Offer weight management — Patient refuses

Patient accepts

3-month weight loss programme, including: exercise; behavioural advice; diet; support scheme (family, health centre, community)

Successful outcome e.g. > 5 kg loss | Unsuccessful outcome

Note: This scheme is for guidance only, but provides a logical management process to be evaluated and modified in each centre. See Table 12 for graded recommendations and supporting evidence for each stage of the scheme.

Maintenance of weight loss is achieved
Regular monitoring
Prevention of further weight gain

Consider specialist referral for surgery if BMI > 35 with major risk factors

Healthy eating advice

Figure 19 *Weight management in primary health care/community.*
(Reproduced with permission of the SIGN.[22])

considered inappropriate to base services in hospitals, which are relatively distant and inaccessible for most patients in their home situations. Many of the tools of management, including investigation and treatment – specifically group counselling and family support – are more readily accessible in a primary care context. Although there is a clear need for centres of specialist excellence – for research, policy development, and the management of specific and unusual clinical problems – the great majority of patients will be better managed in a primary care setting. This assertion itself carries clear resource implications, and the management programme needs to be tested and evaluated before any requirement to provide such a service is made.

The weight-management scheme in *Figure 19* suggests that patients in need of weight management should be obtained from conventional routes, i.e. self-referral of those seeking help and those identified opportunistically as being overweight when they present with related or other health problems. It is also suggested that a practice audit might be appropriate for identifying people who have weight problems developing, with the aim that they should be brought into a structured programme of management before secondary health problems become manifest and start adding to health service costs.

A proportion of patients who should be advised to seek advice about weight gain currently do not regard themselves as having a problem and do not come forward for treatment, or they respond poorly to advice. This mismatch can only be resolved by better health education, conducted at national or local levels. The aim of this health education should be to target overweight individuals who are at the greatest risk of ill health and the waist circumference cut-off points are now being adapted for this purpose.

Goals of weight management

Modern weight management goes a great deal further than slimming or weight loss and involves some negotiating with patients which will result in achieving success in four different ways. Firstly, weight management incorporates *avoiding weight gain* (both in young obesity-prone individuals and in people who have gained and lost weight); secondly, in *losing weight*, where appropriate; thirdly, in the *management of other risk factors* present in people with weight problems, such as smoking, poor diet composition, physical inactivity, adverse plasma lipids and high blood pressure. Finally, the *poor self-esteem* of obese patients needs to be corrected. Successful weight management involves all of these elements, at a clinical level, supported by population-directed health promotion. Baseline assessment is an essential first step for individual patient management and for audit of the service provided.

The goals of management may be couched in terms of weight change or in terms of secondary clinical outcomes *(Table 13)*. In practice, most clinical improvements occur together and evaluation in terms of weight change alone is still of great value.

Recognizing the separate importance of weight loss and weight management, it is logically possible that an effective programme could use different approaches for these components, e.g. a drug for weight loss, and diet and exercise for weight management, or vice versa. It is important that patients should have a clear understanding of the strategy being employed, and that they should have simple and achievable behavioural targets related to regulation of their eating pattern, restriction of fat intake, regular physical activity, quantitative target fruit and vegetable consumption, and landmarks for establishing self-esteem.

This broad view of weight management is new – particularly the emphasis on its value. Organized programmes for weight management have only very recently been recognized as a priority for comprehensive health care. It is a fact that, in industrialized societies adult weights usually increase from the teens to the 50s, and more so for some than for others. Now that the medical hazards and the costs of obesity are clear, the need is apparent to avoid weight gain, preferably before becoming overweight in the first place, but equally after having lost some weight for those who are already running into difficulties. New professional skills are particularly needed by all health professionals, and comprehensive, structured, long-term programmes need to be made attractive and accessible.

Table 13 Appropriate clinical targets for the management of obesity and its complications.

Co-morbidity	Appropriate target
NIDDM and glucose intolerance	Return to normal fasting blood glucose; reduced use of oral hypoglycaemia agents; fall in glycosylated haemoglobin levels
Hypertension	Improvement in blood pressure and reduction in the need for coexisting hypotensive agents
Hyperlipidaemia	Defined improvements in total cholesterol, fasting triglycerides, HDL cholesterol, postprandial lipid clearance
Abdominal fat	Reduced waist measurment
Sleep apnoea	Reduction in sleep apnoea
Arthritis/back pain	Increased mobility; reduced need for drug therapy
Reproductive function	Improved reproductive function with regular menstruation
Psychosocial functioning	Improved quality of life; reduced anxiety; reduced depression; improved social interaction
Exercise intolerance	Improved exercise tolerance; reduced breathlessness

In the past it was usual for doctors and other health professionals to focus on those with severe problems, e.g. with BMI > 30 kg/m^2, with the general aim of reducing weights right down to ideal levels, i.e. to a BMI of 21 kg/m^2, or at least into the acceptable range < 25 kg/m^2. Although most people can lose weight, these targets are almost never reached, so the patients are castigated as failures, or the treatment is dismissed as ineffective. Such conclusions are based on misunderstandings at several levels. Not all patients will achieve the same amount of weight loss but several degrees of success can be identified, remembering that, without intervention, most people will continue to gain weight *(Figure 20)*.

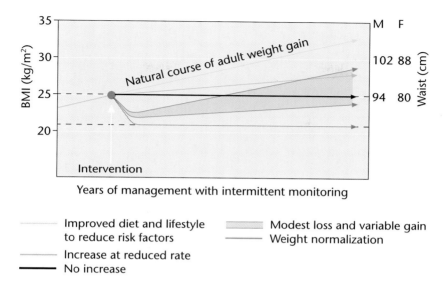

Figure 20 *Possible indicators of success in obesity-management programmes.*

What is practically and theoretically achievable?

A new understanding is needed of the amount of weight loss that is physically possible and practically attainable. Adipose tissue contains lipid (9 kcal/g), but the extra blood supply, fibrous supporting tissue, musculature, etc., means that the energy content of weight loss is ultimately c. 7000 kcal/kg. A patient of 95 kg and an ideal weight of 60 kg would need to shed 35 × 7000 = 245 000 kcal. On a 1000 kcal/day diet, this could be achieved in c. 250 days. Of course, this is theoretically possible and could be achieved by a captive patient fed a precise diet. However, it is highly improbable for a free-living person, and particularly for one with an underlying predisposition for appetite to exceed metabolic need. Experience shows that successful slimmers lose 0.5–1.0 kg/week, and are able to keep this up for 3–6 months at most. This demands a daily dietary restriction of 500–1000 kcal, i.e. sustained major restriction. The end result is a weight loss in the range of c. 5–20 kg. In practice, an average of c. 6–8 kg is achievable, in good centres. These figures justify a target of 10 kg loss and a success criterion of ⩾5 kg.

Weight maintenance could again theoretically be achieved, i.e. static weight after loss by captive patients fed exactly what is needed for weight stability. In practice, weight regain of 2–3 kg/year is common and a modified rate of gain should be considered successful *(Figure 20)*.

What is needed to improve health?

The evidence of benefits of weight loss (see Chapter 5) indicate that most of the health gains from weight loss are achieved with the first 5–10 kg of loss, i.e. restricted by a total of 35 000–70 000 kcal. At 1 kg (7000 kcal)/week, this is achievable in 5–10 weeks on a diet of 1500–2000 kcal. Attempting to lose more weight than this is usually unsuccessful and does not bring important additional health benefits for most patients. Using any method, weight loss is usually complete in 3–4 months. Given the enormous weight of evidence that most people cannot carry on losing weight beyond *c.* 4 months, it is unreasonable, and indeed counterproductive, to expect or to ask them to do so. It is interesting that a loss of 10 kg (22 lb) reduces the metabolic rate by only *c.* 200 kcal/day. For some patients there may be a need to lose more for a specific purpose, such as for the very obese to correct NIDDM or sleep apnoea, before elective abdominal surgery, or when risk factors remain high.

Based on these considerations, i.e. what is practically realistic and what brings health gains, clinical guidelines have proposed that weight loss of > 5 kg (usually *c.* 5%) should be considered successful, especially if risk factors are improved. Loss of > 10 kg is considered very successful. Both of these targets can be attained in a 3–4 month programme. Greater loss, e.g. > 20 kg, requires a long period of *c.* 6 months and should be considered exceptional.

The final target of any weight-management programme is to avoid or minimize weight gain in the long term. This is important both as a primary preventive target and in the management of people who are already overweight, both those who have lost weight and those who have not been able to. A target gain or regain < 3 kg in more than 2 years is considered a reasonable working target. It is not recognized that weight maintenance after weight loss cannot be left to chance, but requires a specific programme incorporating cognitive approaches to raise self-esteem and lifestyle modifications.

Targeting patients at greatest risk

The potential benefits of weight loss, and of avoiding further gain, are maximized when the risks are greatest, e.g. a BMI of > 30 kg/m^2 or a BMI in the range of 25–30 kg/m^2 in the presence of central fat distribution, i.e. waist > 88 cm for women or > 102 cm for men, or when secondary complications such as NIDDM, hyperlipidaemia or hypertension are present, or where a BMI > 25 kg/m^2 is compounded by other risks like smoking. People who fall into these categories can be identified and prioritized for a weight-management programme. In these situations, and perhaps when there is a strong family history of NIDDM or CHD, a more proactive approach should be adopted, by actively recruiting such patients. It is in these situations that the use of drugs should be considered at an earlier stage than otherwise. The benefit/risk ratio for surgical interventions in obesity is considered to become positive when the BMI is > 35 kg/m^2 if secondary complications have already developed, although it can be argued that delaying until this stage may expose the patient to several years of metabolic decompensation as well as to increased postoperative hazards.

As a risk factor for cardiovascular disease, obesity has its greatest influence in young people. Above the age of 60–70 there is no elevation of coronary risk or total mortality from high BMI. Targeting younger overweight people seems justified for coronary prevention. In these older obese adults, however, there seems to be a similar relative risk as in younger people for specific problems such as NIDDM, low HDL cholesterol or hypertension, and relatively major benefits of weight loss may be expected in view of their limited life expectancy. This debate has not yet been resolved, but it seems possible that as people live longer the processes leading to chronic disease are becoming more prominent.

There is, however, a considerable aggravation by age in the common symptoms that accompany obesity *(Table 8)*. Given this, and recognizing in particular the increasing problems of immobility in an ageing population, it would seem prudent to also target the elderly overweight for weight management.

Pregnancy

Weight loss should be avoided in pregnancy for fear of inducing fetal nutrient deficiency or suboptimal intrauterine growth. This anxiety is based partly on the growing evidence that smaller babies have elevated risks of cardiovascular disease in later life, although there is no direct evidence that dietary inadequacy during pregnancy is the reason. It is usually recommended not to become pregnant when actively losing weight, for the same reasons. On the other hand, severe overweight in pregnancy creates a number of obstetric problems, including gestational diabetes and complicated labour. The best plan is to lose weight before conception and then to limit weight gain to reach a BMI of *c.* 28–30 kg/m^2 by term, or to maintain weight if already above this level. Strong advice to breast feed for at least 6 months may help to maximize postpartum weight loss.

chapter 7

Dietary, behavioural and exercise strategies

In simple terms, effective weight management requires that some individuals should spend a period in negative energy balance, i.e. when energy expenditure exceeds energy intake. It also requires the ability to establish and maintain energy balance where energy expenditure equals energy intake for those individuals in whom their appetite would otherwise create a positive energy balance *(Figure 21)*.

The components of energy balance that are modifiable are, on the one hand, food selection and food consumption, and, on the other hand, energy expenditure through voluntary physical activity plus, to some extent, thermogenesis. Although it is possible to consider diet composition as an isolated element, this is not appropriate and, in practice, approaches that rely purely on diet sheets are frustratingly ineffective. Similarly, certain programmes have been devised for weight management that apparently rely entirely on behavioural approaches, addressing attitudes and cognitive issues. In practice, of course, such approaches can only be effective if they lead to greater energy expenditure or to a limitation in energy intake. For these reasons it is not practical or desirable to address these components of energy balance in isolation during weight management, and those involved in this area have, in practice, always used a combination of dietary, behavioural and exercise strategies, adapting these to the individual patient or family.

The conventional approaches to behavioural modification are routinely employed by psychologists. Some approaches known to be

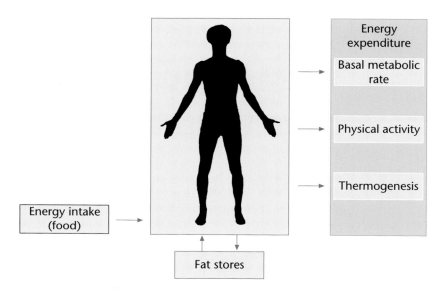

Figure 21 *Energy balance shown schematically. A person will remain weight stable when energy intake equals energy expenditure. A change in fat stores can only result from a change in energy intake, energy output, or both.*

effective in weight management, such as reception of messages, reinforcement of messages, reward systems, partner or 'buddy' systems for support, have all been employed and all have some value. One of the most effective approaches, used in certain commercial organizations, is to formalize the behavioural aspect into a form of contingency contracting such that the counsellor enters a quasi-legal agreement with the patient, who undertakes to take on certain behaviour for a defined period of time. This agreement can be signed by both parties and by a witness, who might be the partner or 'buddy' who is going to provide local policing or support to the patient. For some patients, providing financial incentives to achieve change can be effective, at least for achieving weight loss; however, it is not clear whether this type of approach is of such value in long-term weight maintenance. To be effective the amount of money involved must be large: research has shown that if different payments are made for the same weight-loss programme, those who pay most lose most – even if the money is ultimately to be returned. This type of approach is, of course, inappropriate in a nationalized health service context, although no-loss schemes can be devised, e.g. a patient can undertake to set aside a monthly sum into the safekeeping of an account that would be redeemable either on termination of the programme or on achievement of agreed targets.

A number of studies have compared approaches to weight management using individual one-to-one counselling methods, or group approaches. In general, the results of group methods have proved to be at least as effective as, and in many cases more effective than, individual one-to-one counselling. A group or class approach may not be acceptable to every patient but, where resources are limited, the very large savings that can be made in professional time and resources by using this method make it an attractive proposition. This approach is recommended as the preferred starting point for a weight management programme in the SIGN guidelines designed by the Royal Colleges in Scotland. Although many dieticians and some practice nurses have already begun to use group approaches, this is an unusual approach for disease management in most medical sectors. It is important that the medical backing and support for the scheme is appropriate to the seriousness of the condition. Group management can be effective but specific training in leading groups is required. As a general rule, it is difficult to sustain groups for longer than a few months without repetition, boredom or loss of morale. Attempts to convert therapeutic disease management groups into self-sustaining patient-led groups have been followed in some areas, but data are not available from which to assess their effectiveness. This does, however, seem a logical approach to lifestyle management. The opportunity to link with existing services outside the directly medical sphere (exercise classes, rambling groups, evening class groups, etc.) have not been fully explored, although some general practices in the UK are now prescribing commercially run exercise classes for other patient groups, e.g. in cardiac rehabilitation following myocardial infarction.

Diet modification

It is vital that dietary guidance should be given by confident, trained professionals with the backing and support of doctors. It is insufficient and inappropriate for patients to be 'given a diet' or less still to be 'given a diet sheet'. Taking a holistic view of their health hazards, and of the long-term reduction of elevated risks after weight has stabilized after loss, people with weight problems firstly need professional advice about a healthy balanced diet pattern. In keeping with dietary targets for general health, this should start with advice to take at least five portions of fruit and vegetables daily, and to minimize the amount of saturated fat, i.e. fat from animal sources, in the diet. The major nutrients that provide calories (fat, protein and carbohydrates) have different properties *(Table 14)*. People with weight problems tend to eat rather too

Table 14 Characteristics of macronutrients. Fat appears to be the key macronutrient that undermines the body's weight-regulatory systems, since it is very poorly regulated at the level of both consumption and oxidation.

	Fat	*Protein*	*Carbohydrate*	*Alcohol*
Ability to bring eating to an end	Low	High	Intermediate	Opposite
Ability to suppress hunger	Low	High	High	Stimulating
Contribution to daily energy intake	High	Low	High	Varies
Energy density	High	Low	Low	High
Storage capacity in body	High	None	Low	None
Metabolic pathway to transfer excess intake to another compartment	No	Yes	Yes	Yes
Autoregulation (ability to stimulate own oxidation on intake)	Poor	Good	Good	Poor
Calories per gram	9	4	3.75	7

much fat and too little starchy carbohydrate. Overweight people often still believe, incorrectly, that starch and carbohydrate are 'fattening'. In fact, it is fat that is most fattening, given that it contains 9 kcal/g, compared to 3.75 kcal/g in carbohydrates and 4 kcal/g in protein, so it is safe to maintain, or even to have more, of the nutritious bulky and filling foods such as bread, potatoes, pasta and rice, while cutting down on or cutting out the spreads or sauces that go with them.

The simplistic approach of giving a patient a diet concentrates solely on foods but neglects the complexity of eating patterns. It is now useful to consider giving advice on:

- What you eat
- When you eat
- Where you eat
- With whom you eat
- How you eat

Avoiding totally full-fat milk and dairy products (preferring reduced-fat versions), processed meat products like sausages and pies, and biscuits and baked foods should become a new way of life. This style of eating, relatively high in carbohydrate and low in fat (particularly saturated fat), should be continued after weight loss has ceased. People with weight problems will always have weight problems and this is an important way to help them control their weight. On its own, changing diet composition may not lead to major weight loss, but a low-fat lifestyle does limit further gain and, importantly, also improves cardiovascular risk. One large study[23] showed that switching to low fat foods (without trying to lose weight) led people to consume about 200–400 kcal/day less. This is enough to prevent most weight gain and potentially almost abolish obesity.

In attempts to achieve weight loss, the old fashioned approach was to use calorie-restricted diets, such as 1000–2000 kcal/day. These diets were applied to patients rather indiscriminately. Whilst, in principle, this type of diet will produce weight loss in all overweight people, it has not been seen to be effective. The up-to-date approach is to design 'energy-deficit' diets for individual patients based upon individual energy

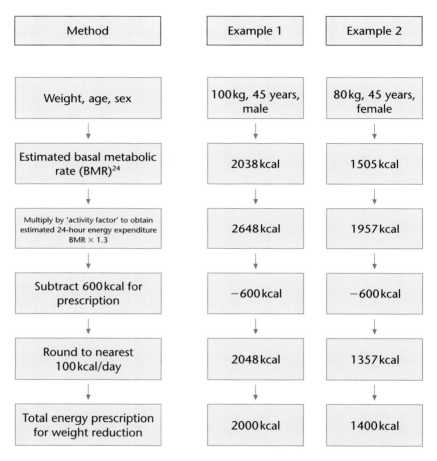

Figure 22 Designing the energy content of a diet for weight loss of 0.5–1 kg/week, assuming a mainly sedentary lifestyle.

requirements. This can be done rather simply using an estimate of the 24-hour BMR (measured in kcal/24 hours), from which a figure of say 600 kcal/day is subtracted. Weight loss of 0.5–1.0 kg per week will result.

This type of approach, using an algorithm *(Figure 22)*, has been found to be very effective in large multicentre trials and comparisons with conventional 1200 kcal diets have been favourable. One such comparison found that the prescription of individual diets with an average of

1600 kcal actually produced a greater weight loss than giving a controlled group of patients a standard 1200 kcal diet, but the main value of the energy-deficit approach is that patients are more likely to be able to adhere to advice and thus to optimize nutrient composition of the diet. On more restrictive, conventional diets, patients rarely adhere to the exact amounts prescribed and may end up overeating inappropriate foods. A relatively small (undeclared) fat intake can easily provide all the calories the patient was supposed not to be eating! It is therefore important to match the calorie content of diets to the individual requirements of patients and to set a level that is achievable over a 3–4 month period of weight loss. The aim is to lose fat, which being very energy dense is lost more slowly than other tissues *(Table 15)*.

Reviews of the literature have shown that patients who embark on weight-loss programmes continue for a variable length of time: the majority, in a well-organized and supportive study, can continue to lose weight for 3–4 months, after which time weight loss tails off; the average weight loss in this time is of the order of 7–10 kg. A very small number of individuals can maintain a weight-loss diet for 6 months and during this time they will lose something of the order of 20 kg. With the aim of achieving the greatest benefit for the most patients, it is now recommended that programmes of weight management should aim for an

Table 15 Approximate calorie contents of nutrients and body tissues.

Nutrient	Calories (kcal/kg)
Fat (lipid)	9000
Alcohol	7000
Protein	4000
Carbohydrate	3750
Dietary fibre	2000–3000
Adipose tissue	7000
Lean muscle	1000

achievable target of say 5–10 kg of weight loss over 3–4 months. Five kilograms weight loss would be considered good and a 10 kg weight loss excellent. This rate of weight loss demands an energy deficit of 500–1000 kcal/day over a period of months. The perceived benefits are small, and much support and encouragement is needed. Any patient who continues to lose 20 kg or more over 6 months would be considered exceptional. If patients lose weight more rapidly, then there is a risk that they are losing disproportionate amounts of muscle (only 1000 kcal/kg). It is important to maintain physical activity to preserve muscle mass.

Following the period of weight loss, usually after about 3 months, it is essential that the comprehensive weight-management programme then takes on board the needs of weight maintenance, which are rather different to those of weight loss. It is at this stage that the patient and their family need very clear explanations of the principles involved and of the targets in weight maintenance. A proposed target is that the patient should regain < 3 kg of that which has been lost over a period of 2 years or more. It has to be recognized that weight does tend to increase in adults up to about the age of 60, so some weight gain in people who have lost weight is probably not unreasonable, providing that they do not return to the level that they would have reached without any intervention *(Figure 20)*. These concepts and their practical application are largely new to health professionals, and they will certainly be unusual to most patients who have been accustomed to calls to lose weight and then to lose more weight. *It is important to regard weight maintenance as a success, even in people with weight problems who have lost little weight.*

Children

The problem of obesity in children is rather different from that in adults and separate guidelines have been published.[25] The potential risks from weight loss in this age group are uncertain. The recognition that there may be hazards for physical and psychological development from weight loss during childhood has led to the recommendation that, in most situations, weight loss should not be a target in the weight management of children. Because of the risks of stigmatization, and in view of the results of interventions, family-based approaches are to be preferred, with a focus on overall lifestyle *(Figure 23)*. The proposed goal is that overweight children should be encouraged to limit weight gain such that their BMI proceeds to the interval marked by the lines on the

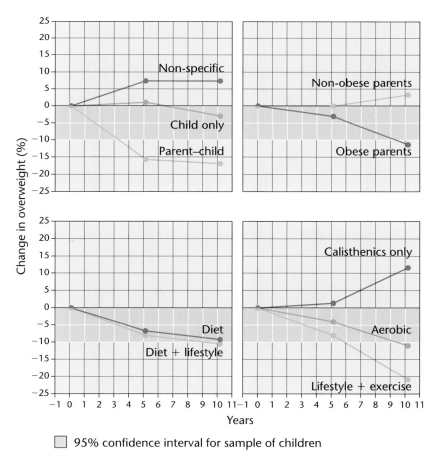

95% confidence interval for sample of children

Figure 23 *Changes in percentage overweight after 5 and 10 years follow-up for obese children randomly assigned to 10 interventions across four studies. (Reproduced with permission from Epstein et al.[26])*

charts shown in *Appendix A* over a 2–3 year period. Weight management for children should always be a family-directed exercise, concentrating on diet composition for health and on physical activity. It should be recognized that overweight in children under the age of 10 does not necessarily proceed to obesity in adulthood. However, overweight teenagers unfortunately do usually track through age to become overweight adults. Children from the age of 10 are weight conscious and also adaptable in terms of eating habits and lifestyle, so results can be rewarding. Amongst older teenagers, it is usually preferable to deal directly with the child, rather than through the parents.

Food and eating behaviour

Food and eating are central features in the identity of individuals, families and entire cultures. What we choose to eat and how we eat it are moulded by generations of cultural exposure, and to imagine that these things can be changed in response to a set of simple instructions is naïve. On the other hand, food and eating habits do change. Indeed, individual experience indicates that there have been remarkable changes even over a 10–20 year period. Perhaps one of the most striking societal changes has been the adoption (and acceptance) of between-meal snacking, nibbling or grazing. This habit has been related to the development and wide promotion of a completely new range of easily stored, ready-to-eat snacks (often high in sugar and fat), which can be related to the rising prevalence of obesity. Thus, people do change food habits and eating patterns – but not overnight. National breakfast habits have changed, but only through immense commercial marketing. In principle, a similar lay communication approach could be harnessed for health. Already the 'five-a-day' message for fruit and vegetables has become very widely known, and people are clearly starting to adopt this behaviour, which is probably the most important single step towards health and weight management.

Behavioural modification

A number of behavioural approaches have been developed for different purposes. Various psychological/behavioural models of food choice are commonly discussed. These include the Stages of Change model of Prochasta and di Clemente,[27] which was originally, and most usefully, applied to addictions (*Figure 24*). In principle, a patient's readiness to change behaviour defines how successful they are likely to be. Efforts to generate change should be limited to those who are ready, and be followed by maintenance. Although in principle self-fulfilling, this approach has not been so effective with weight management as with addiction breaking, where only one behaviour is targeted and needs to be stopped. Another more involved model is the Theory of Reasoned Action of Fishbein and Ajzen (*Figure 25*).[28] This has been of some use in explaining behaviour and may identify influential factors. Again, however, the value in managing individual obese patients is uncertain.

Newer approaches include motivational interview and cognitive behaviour therapy. To some extent, both approaches merely formalize what experienced doctors and dietitians have already been doing in an unstructured way – focusing on giving value to achievable gains.

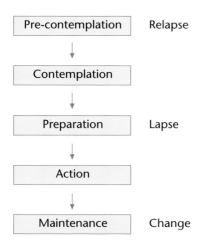

Figure 24 *Stages of change model. (From Prochasta and DiClemente.[27])*

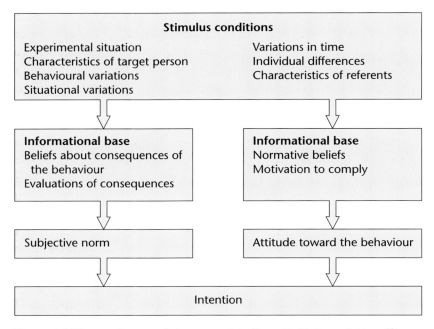

Figure 25 *Theory of reasoned change model. (From Fishbein and Ajzen.[28])*

If eating habits are to change, the entire process of food choice, acquisition and consumption must be addressed. To change their shopping pattern, patients must not buy what is not needed, so a planned approach should be encouraged, using shopping lists and eating plans or menus. Examples can initially be provided by a therapist, but the patient soon has to take responsibility for their day-to-day shopping. People with weight problems often have rather undisciplined eating and a lot can be achieved by sticking to simple rules about meals. A useful start is for patients to complete a diary of food and eating habits for 14 days, which many then use to scrutinize and modify their diets. A diary is also useful for dieticians, as it can be analysed using a food database – a process which has been simplified by systems such as rapid data entry using barcodes. However, the main value of therapy or counselling is more to do with the style of eating, the pattern of meals and the reason why a particular choice was made, or is regularly made. It is therefore valuable to have information about the context of eating, as well as the content of meals or snacks. It seems that snacking in the evenings is a very common problem – often while watching television. The internal cue which leads to that eating may in fact be a result of inactivity and boredom. The body may just need a change, such as getting up, going outside and walking for 5–10 minutes; the apparent 'hunger' may then recede.

Firm advice to have three meals a day and no snacks in between may be needed before trying to modify dietary components. A breakfast such as porridge is filling and nutritious but low in calories, and is often effective in reducing appetite later. Porridge and breakfast cereals are also useful at other times of the day rather than snacking on biscuits and other high-calorie foods. Offering practical guidance increases credibility, e.g. suggest tips such as making an extra bowl of porridge in the morning which can be kept in the fridge and then heated in a microwave to be eaten as a low-calorie bedtime snack. Bread is also nutritious and relatively low in calories, but people with weight problems can usefully decide to forego all butter or margarine whilst attempting to lose weight. It is the spreads that provide most calories per mouthful and this needs to be reflected in shopping lists. Fruit and vegetables, as mentioned earlier, should add up to at least five portions (each apple-sized, *c.* 80 g) per day. These foods are filling, refreshing, rich in micronutrients but low in calories. To eat five portions a day, however, does demand a change in shopping, as these foods need to be bought at least twice a week.

Agreeing to eat only off a plate, and never to eat with the fingers, is often effective. This may overcome temptation in places like petrol stations and corner shops, as well as avoiding unplanned between-meal eating. However, rules of these kinds are only successful if the patient agrees to enforce them. Details need to be discussed and negotiated, and then reviewed or renegotiated. Rewards and incentives are effective in behavioural therapy, and a non-food reward system is valuable for improving compliance. Recruiting a partner or 'buddy' to confide in and serve as a local 'policeman/woman' often improves results. In some settings, formal legal-style agreements can be signed by the patient, declaring agreed rules for a set period, and countersigned by the partner who undertakes to help maintain the agreement.

Box 1 shows a checklist of behavioural approaches which can be considered with every patient. Not all will be effective for everyone and offering a 'menu' of changes can be educational as well as effective.

Box 1 Prioritised health aims for behavioural approaches in weight management.

- Become a non-smoker (top priority)
- Eat at least five portions of fruit and vegetables daily
- Eat fish at least twice a week
- 20–30 minutes moderate activity daily (to breathe hard or break sweat)
- Avoid future weight gain (before and after loss)
- Achieve weight loss of 5–10 kg in three-month stages
- Feel proud to have accomplished each of these

Physical activity

Although obese people undertake less voluntary exercise than people of normal weight, the effort required is much greater. Most people with a BMI > 30 kg/m^2 simply cannot exercise more, and they risk damage to joints and muscles if they do. Furthermore, it is very difficult to lose weight by increasing exercise or physical activity alone. Remembering that each kilogram of adipose tissue (fat) contains *c.* 7000 kcal; therefore, 7 kg (about a stone) contains *c.* 50 000 kcal. It would take years to burn off this number of calories from the type of extra physical exercise that overweight people can take, even if they manage it daily. On the other hand, the advantages of physical activity are enormous in helping people to feel better, in overcoming depression, in reducing blood cholesterol and blood pressure, and in reducing the risks of diabetes, and also in reducing appetite in the long term.

Increasing physical activity is vital for weight maintenance and to avoid weight gain, and it also helps to protect valuable muscle when people are losing weight, i.e. to promote the loss of fat *(Box 2)*. The metabolic rate of a patient who has lost 7 kg (15 lb) will be reduced by *c.* 120 kcal/day: to maintain this lower weight, the patient must either eat 120 kcal/day less (equivalent to two biscuits) or take *c.* 20 minutes/day of gentle activity (e.g. brisk walking) to burn off the 120 kcal. In a structured programme for health and weight management, a good start is to trade food for movement, e.g. to walk about a little instead of sitting down for coffee and biscuits. A creative solution is to agree, perhaps for a trial period of 6 weeks (or 12 weeks), to eat no biscuits or other snacks between meals. Instead, go outside and walk around the building for at least 10 minutes, and then have a cup of tea. Trying different varieties of tea can increase the interest and sustainability of this advice.

Box 2 Proposed mechanisms linking exercise with the success of weight maintenance. (Adapted from Saris.[29])

- Increased energy expenditure
- Improvement of body composition
  - Fat loss
  - Preservation of lean body mass
  - Reduction of visceral fat deposit
- Increased capacity for fat mobilization and oxidation
- Control of food intake
  - Short-term reduction of appetite
  - Reduction of fat intake
- Prevents leptin entry into brain
- Stimulation of thermogenic response
  - Resting metabolic rate
  - Diet-induced thermogenesis
- Change in muscle morphology and biochemical capacity
- Increased insulin sensitivity
- Improved plasma lipid and lipoprotein profile
- Reduced blood pressure
- Better aerobic fitness
- Positive psychological effects

The sort of activities to be considered by the overweight are opportunistic: using stairs or steps instead of lifts of escalators; walking for all journeys less than, say, 1 mile, or deciding to walk for a least 1 mile into and back from work (e.g. getting off the bus early or getting on to it later); introducing at least one television-free day per week and then increasing the number of television-free days.

Self-esteem and confidence

It is increasingly clear that low self-esteem and poor confidence, so common in the obese, are real impediments to taking charge of a life problem like obesity. Self-esteem usually improves with weight loss if the hard work and extent of self-denial is recognized and praised. It is also possible to break the vicious cycle by addressing self-esteem directly. Classes are run by clinical psychologists in some areas and may have a value.

Any new leisure activity is worth considering – walking, jogging and/or swimming may all be appropriate for some patients. These activities often include a social and psychological dimension as well as the purely physical. Joining a group or evening class to enjoy a new social life will inevitably increase the physical activity a little, but it may be more important for obese patients to explore new skills in a non-competitive environment. This has added value, since boredom, often confused with depression, is a common factor in the overweight. Not all patients will be amenable to all these measures, but intervention approaches help some of them.

Expected rate of weight loss

Many people attempting to lose weight have come unstuck, and many doctors and other health professionals have lost credibility, by failing to understand the rate at which weight can be lost. Management expectations in the doctor–patient relationship is therefore crucial for success.

Since each kilogram of adipose tissue contains *c.* 7000 kcal, a very strict diet, cutting back by 500 kcal/day, will lead to weight loss of *c*. 0.5 kg (1 lb)/week – a loss of 7 kg (15 lb) in *c*. 3 months. A faster weight loss of up to 1 kg/week can be achieved, but only by a minority of people and for a fairly short period. On average, most people who follow sensible dietary advice can lose 5–10 kg in a period of 2–3 months. *Fast rates of weight loss, as well as being difficult to sustain, can be dangerous, since they often imply excessive loss of muscle or other body tissue.*

As a general rule, weight loss of 0.5 kg (1 lb)/week is good and 1 kg (2 lb)/week excellent – anything more than this is potentially dangerous. Bathroom scales do not give a good guide to weight loss, since body water can change quite markedly, particularly in women. It is possible to lose 1 kg of fat in a week through hard work sticking to a diet but to gain 1.5 kg in water temporarily. The bathroom scales would show weight gain over this period and this can be very demoralizing. A simple guide to weight loss is a reduction in waist circumference. The aim is for a reduction in the waist circumference of *c*. 5–10 cm in 2–3 months. After weight loss for 3 months, it is usually not a good plan to try to continue to lose weight immediately. The best plan is to learn how to maintain the new lower weight for a period of time before trying to lose more. *Patients need continued support and encouragement for weight mainte-nance, and one of the best predictors of success is the frequency of professional contact. Accurate weighing and measurement of the waist circumference provide a very positive contact.*

chapter 8

The role of drug therapy

The pharmacotherapy of obesity has been a source of serious confusion in the past. Within some branches of the medical profession there remains serious ignorance, which has ultimately led to some widely-publicized unscrupulous practitioners prescribing to a frustrated patient group which deserves better understanding and service.

Certain drugs that have often been used in attempts to lose weight should *never* be prescribed as a treatment for obesity. Oedema in the overweight or obese usually reflects a local problem in the legs and is not the result of sodium retention, and it responds poorly to diuretics. The use of diuretics in overweight women is strongly associated with 'cyclical' oedema, whose solution usually lies in weight loss and not in drug therapy. Amphetamines undoubtedly reduce appetite but they, and other functionally-related drugs, have centrally stimulating addictive properties with abuse potential, and may cause hypertensive crises. They are controlled drugs and should never be used for weight management. In the past, a number of drugs developed for weight loss, like fenfluramine and phentermine, had structural similarities to amphetamines, but different pharmacologies, lacking the mood-altering and addictive properties. They have been withdrawn over other concerns about safety.

The ideal drug for weight management would reduce energy intake, increase energy expenditure and improve risk factors for obesity-related conditions *(Box 3)*. One approach to reducing appetite, or to promoting the feeling of satiety after eating a meal, is by increasing the neurotrans-

Box 3 Characteristics of an ideal energy balance regulator to manage obesity.

- Demonstrated effect on reducing body weight and weight-dependent disease*
- Tolerable and/or transient side effects
- No addictive properties
- A maintained efficacy when used long term
- No major problems after years of administration
- Known mechanisms of action(s)
- A reasonable cost
- Possible to identify responders at an early stage in treatement

*Note that drug approval agencies such as the US FDA require a minimum of 5% additional weight loss over that which is achieved by a placebo-treatment regimen

mitters 5-hydroxy-tryptamine, also known as serotonin or 5-HT, noradrenaline and dopamine in the brain.

Sibutramine, offers the potential advantage of having both serotonin and noradrenaline reuptake inhibition (SRNI) activity, and so two complementary mechanisms for producing satiety. It is also mildly thermogenic by central effects which attenuates the usual decline in metabolic rate with weight loss. It thus earns the title of an energy balance regulator. The side-effect profiles are good. Since sibutramine has no significant effect on dopaminergic systems, it is not addictive and has no abuse potential. The main effect in humans is to delay the reappearance of hunger or prolong the pleasant feeling of fullness after a meal, and so reduces the need for snacks between meals. Because snacks tend to be high in fat, consumption of fat, and therefore calories, falls.

In animal studies, sibutramine may be selective in reducing appetite for carbohydrate because of a specific hypothalamic action of serotonin. There is no evidence for selective carbohydrate-intake appetite suppression in humans. A proportion of patients on sibutramine do not lose weight and they can be identified as those who will fail to lose 2 kg within the first 4 months of treatment. If these patients are excluded then a weight loss of 8–10 kg can be expected, on average, maintained for at least 2 years. The best results with sibutramine have come from studies where this drug is used together with diet and exercise plans when the patient knows they are getting this active drug. The large STORM trial[30] achieved 12 kg weight loss, which was extremely well maintained for 2 years (*Figure 26*). Sibutramine was able to maintain similar weight loss after initial VLCD treatment. Sibutramine is remarkably free from worrying side effects and all the associated risk factors of obesity improve with weight loss on this drug. However, blood pressure does not decline as much as it would from the same degree of weight loss without its use, which reflects the sympathetic action of sibutramine; it also produces a small increase in the pulse rate, of around 3–4 beats/minute, about the same as salbutamol.

Sibutramine was first developed as a potential SRNI antidepressant. Its serotoninergic and noradrenergic effects may be shared, to some extent, by other drugs in this group of SRNI marketed as antidepressants, e.g. paroxetine, fluoxetine, venlafaxine and sertraline, however, these drugs have not been shown to produce comparable weight loss.

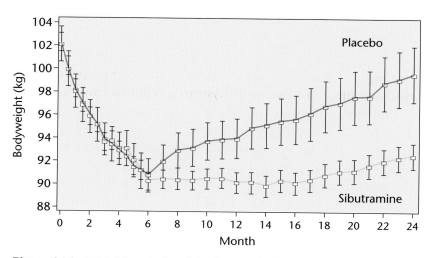

Figure 26 STORM: Mean bodyweight changes during weight loss and weight maintenance phases over 2 years (Observed data).[30]

Ephedrine/caffeine

The ephedrine/caffeine combination is favoured in Denmark and some other countries. These two products are both plant derived and have separate effects to increase energy expenditure and reduce appetite, based on a sympathetic system, with the potential for dose-related unwanted sympathetic effects such as hypertension, agitation and sleeplessness. However, this approach is acceptable to many patients, and well sustained weight losses of 5–10 kg have been reported

Orlistat

The lipase inhibitor orlistat (tetrahydrolipostatin) was developed to reduce the absorption of fat from the small intestine, resulting in mild steatorrhoea and the wastage of fat calories from food by preventing their absorption. Orlistat will produce unacceptable steatorrhoea if the diet is high in fat, but provided that <30% of energy comes from fat it has been found to be acceptable. Indeed, patients may not know if they are on orlistat or placebo if they follow dietetic advice. If patients can lose 2.5 kg on a low-fat diet alone and then succeed in losing 5% of body weight within 12 weeks on orlistat, then they can expect to lose 16% of body weight on average and to maintain that weight loss for at least 1 year. This success was found in only one-third of patients entering clinical trials, but the improvement in metabolic risk factors was very striking, and maintained for at least 2 years (*Figure 27*). There is improvement in all the risk factors associated with obesity, the lipid-lowering effect being enhanced by fat malabsorption. Because orlistat is not absorbed by the gut, side effects are rare, other than looseness of stools if patients fail to follow the low fat diet. There may be concern if patients have marginal or low intakes of vitamins, but this was not a problem in clinical trials. Several agents under research are intended to increase thermogenesis.

Various weight management drugs are listed in *Table 16*.

Table 16 Weight-management drugs currently available for use or under development.

Principal mode of action	Drug name
Centrally acting	
Noradrenergic	Phentermine
Combined serotonergic and noradrenergic reuptake inhibitor	Sibutramine
Leptin receptor agonist	Leptin analogues
Peripherally acting	
Lipase inhibitor	Orlistat (tetrahydrolipostatin)
Peripherally and centrally acting	
Thermogenic and anorectic	Ephedrine/caffeine

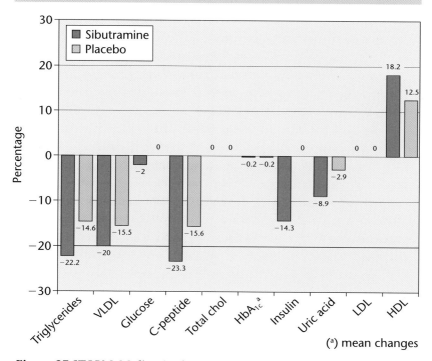

Figure 27 *STORM: Median % change in metabolic risk factors at 2 years from baseline for sibutramine and placebo patients (Observed data).*[33]

Using drugs for weight management

There is no drug which, on its own, can safely overcome human appetite. On their own, or combined with a diet, the currently available drugs from a range of classes will lead to extra weight loss (i.e. above that with placebo) of *c.* 2–3 kg (8 lb) on average. As with most drugs in other fields of medicine, a proportion of patients, *c.* 1 in 5, do not respond to these drugs at all and should have their treatment changed after 4–8 weeks if weight has not fallen by 2 kg. The rest can expect to lose a mean of 7–10 kg from the drug and dietary advice combined. The weight loss for responders is therefore rather better than in the whole-treatment group of a placebo-controlled clinical trial. Isolated individuals have exaggerated responses, losing 20 kg or more. The search for more potent weight loss should be tempered by concern for such individuals, and the focus should in future be on maintaining weight.

The use of drug therapy just for short periods, e.g. 3 months, is of doubtful value unless the weight loss can be maintained, either by continuing the drug or by some other means. This does not necessarily justify lifelong therapy but few interventions, other than surgery, can consistently limit weight regain after loss.

Perhaps more important than the initial help with weight loss, drugs can overcome appetite of the order of 150 kcal/day, which, as discussed above, is enough to maintain a body weight that has been reduced by 5–10 kg (15 lb) by any approach. Although the outcomes of very long-term trials are currently unavailable, it appears that the drugs remain effective as long as they are taken with a weight-maintaining dietary regimen up to at least 2 years. On withdrawal, weight tends to increase. Their main role for pharmacotherapy in the future may, in fact, be to help maintain weight loss by taking them indefinitely, rather than just to achieve weight loss over a short period of time. A major aim of using drugs for long-term weight management is to reduce the need for other drugs that often need to be prescribed for complications of obesity, such as analgesics for arthritis, lipid-lowering drugs, antihypertensive drugs and oral hypoglycaemic agents. Because of the chronic or even permanent nature of the medical consequences, all of these drugs are usually taken indefinitely. Obviously, to be used in this way in younger people, who have not yet developed medical consequences of long-term obesity, drugs will have to be very safe.

A major medical concern over safety has been the link between serotonin-releasing agents and the rare condition of primary pulmonary hypertension (PPH). This is a very rare condition, with a mortality rate of 50%, affecting about one in half a million people annually. In the 1960s, an association was made with a serotonin-releasing agent no longer on the market (aminorex fumarate) and increasing numbers of cases were linked with dexfenfluramine. This problem was aggravated by combination with phentermine, which has monoamine oxidase (MAO) inhibitory action. PPH has not been linked with serotonin reuptake inhibitors like sibutramine.

Some of the drug-related cases have resolved with drug withdrawal, but the links with drugs have been difficult to establish with certainty because PPH is also linked with obesity *per se* and with smoking. Most reported cases were in obese French women, who are often inclined to smoke in misguided attempts to control their appetite. Fenfluramine and dexfenfluramine were withdrawn by the manufacturers in 1997, following publication of some uncontrolled case reports suggesting a link with valvular heart disease – almost all in-patients treated with a combination of fenfluramine and phentermine in the USA. This was despite the apparent safe use of fenfluramine and dexfenfluramine in many millions of patients for over 20 years in other countries. Subsequent research has indicated that subclinical value dysfunction is common in obesity, and probably not aggravated by anti-obesity drugs.

The role of drugs in weight management was the subject of a report from the Royal College of Physicians, London.[31] On the basis of available evidence before the withdrawal of dexfenfluramine, it was thought prudent to restrict use to patients with BMI > 30 kg/m^2 for a period of 12 months. As a matter of principle, drugs are only recommended after a 3-month period of diet and exercise. The guidelines do not yet differentiate between the potentially separate roles of drugs for initiating weight loss and for maintaining weight in the long term. It is, however, recommended that use should only be continued if there is a 10% weight loss at 3 months. This criterion is reasonable for patients weighing < 90–100 kg, but is unreasonable and potentially dangerous for very overweight patients – 10% of 200 kg is 20 kg loss and this would be a worrying target. Future guidelines will need to consider this point.

It is likely that, with better clinical trials evidence, future guidelines will be able to make recommendations separately for initiating weight loss and for maintaining body weight to prevent gain. It may be possible to set more reasoned criteria on which to detect non-responders to drug therapy. For example, those who fail to lose 2 kg in 4 weeks are very unlikely to lose weight subsequently and the drug should be stopped.

As better evidence is published, it is becoming more acceptable to use anti-obesity drugs in patients with lower BMI (e.g. > 27 kg/m^2) who have the greatest health risks, e.g. cardiovascular disease or arthritis threatening mobility. This is already reflected in the licensed indication for sibutramine and orlistat in both the USA and Europe. Better evidence in very obese subjects, e.g. BMI > 50 kg/m^2, is needed in order to give evidence-based recommendations for these patients, but there are no upper BMI limits to prescription.

There have been recent calls for long-term trials to look at the impact of drug therapy for weight loss on hard end points such as myocardial infarction or death. It is certainly possible, and theoretically likely, that substantial weight loss will reduce myocardial infarction and delay death. The reason for such a trial would be to establish whether some factor associated with the drug itself might interfere with the benefits to be expected from weight loss. There are very major problems from a conceptual and practical point of view about conducting trials of this kind. Patients who volunteer for weight-loss trials are likely to be those who will lose weight anyway and so maintaining a placebo or untreated group for many years is a practical impossibility. There is also an important theoretical point which is often misunderstood. The treatment which will reduce heart disease and mortality is, in fact, weight loss, whereas the prescription might be that for a drug plus diet and exercise. In any drug trial of this kind, there will be a range of weight losses, extending from no loss at all in some patients to major weight loss, perhaps 20 kg, in other patients. The range of weight changes in a control group is very similar with a great deal of overlap. An alternative experimental design to address this problem would be to evaluate the impact of weight loss on myocardial infarction or long-term mortality using a regression analysis, and perhaps using a menu of active treatment from which it would be possible to identify the benefits of weight loss itself and variations in any impacts between the effects of weight loss achieved by different means. With any drug treatment in weight management, the major intervention is diet and exercise, with the drug aiding compliance with these measures. For this reason, results of open trials are often greater than those in the placebo-controlled study, and patients have less faith in the tablet and are less likely to comply with dietary and lifestyle measures.

An important feature of the guidelines for drug use was the requirement that the patient's general practitioner should be informed of the prescription, to avoid confusion or multiple prescriptions being collected. Obesity treatment has long been a lucrative activity for unscrupulous practitioners and many have been taken to court, e.g. for prescribing drugs to patients who are not overweight, or doing so without adequate documentation and follow-up. Communicating with general practitioners would usually avoid this.

Box 4 Possible goals of drug therapy for obesity.

- Weight loss
  - More loss
  - Faster loss
  - More people succeed
- Weight maintenance
- Reduce symptoms
- Restrict secondary disorders
- Improve life expectancy

chapter 9

Surgery for obesity

Some people with severe obesity are simply unable to control their appetite to limit food intake in the long term sufficiently well to control their weight adequately. When there are serious weight problems coupled with medical complications, the risks of premature mortality and the personal burden of ill health from continuing obesity are so great that surgery to the stomach is justifiable from an analysis of clinical risks and benefits.

In general, a surgical approach is limited to those with a BMI >35 kg/m². Any abdominal surgery is quite a major undertaking and, in addition, is likely to be more complicated for people who have serious weight problems. It is therefore vital that every effort should be made to lose weight before surgery, and this may include temporary measures such as a very-low-calorie diet and tooth-wiring. Nutritional status may need to be ensured by prescribing micronutrient supplements in amounts equivalent to daily requirements for healthy individuals. The operation most widely used in Europe is gastroplication or gastric stapling *(Figure 28)*, which effectively reduces the size of the stomach so that it is able to accommodate only *c.* 50 ml. To avoid early breakdown of the staple line after this operation, patients have to consume a liquid-only diet for *c.* 3 months, supplemented with iron and vitamins, and then, under dietetic supervision, move onto a carefully balanced diet taken in small amounts of food throughout the day. As a less intrusive alternative, a gastric 'banding' laparoscopic method has been developed.

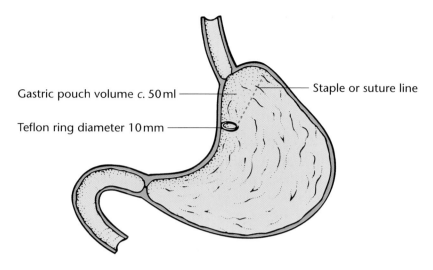

Gastric pouch volume *c.* 50 ml

Teflon ring diameter 10 mm

Staple or suture line

Figure 28 *Diagram of vertical banded gastroplication. Cholescystectomy is usually performed simultaneously.*

More recently gastric bypass surgery is also gaining support and good success rates have been published in the USA. An alternative operation which is gaining favour is gastric bypass. This produces greater and more sustained weight loss, but with the common hazard of introducing a dumping syndrome.

Following these types of operations, patients usually lose *c.* 30–70 kg (70–150 lb) over 12–18 months, and the medical complications of obesity, such as NIDDM, usually disappear. The development of diabetes or hypertension is virtually abolished and hypertension is much improved, although it can develop later. One of the most rewarding subsequent benefits is a reduction in anxiety or depression, despite the demands made on social aspects of eating. It achieves nothing that could not be achieved, in theory at least, by the same changes in diet without going through an operation. On the other hand, it is highly effective, and predictably so. A very large Swedish study[32] has shown that gastroplication results in dramatically improved qualities of life and reductions in major health hazards.

When an impasse is reached, with conservative methods failing to achieve weight loss or health improvement, and the patient fulfils the criteria for surgery, and agrees to or requests it, the patient will be advised to see a psychologist or psychiatrist to explore the behavioural, psychological and social consequences. This type of surgery has very definite perioperative risks, particularly of serious postoperative infections, and carries a mortality risk of up to 1%. Cholecystectomy is usually performed simultaneously to avoid the common problem of gallstones during rapid weight loss. Access to a high-dependency unit for ventilatory support is desirable. Postoperative medical, dietetic and possible psychiatric support will be required for life.

Debate about the cost effectiveness of obesity surgery is now carefully examining long-term results. It appears that weight loss up to 2 years is good by any current method. In the longer term, weight regain is usual after gastroplication or banding, presumably because the patient's appetite remains high and they find ways to increase caloric intake by liquidizing foods, etc. Endoscopy rarely shows expansion of the gastric pouch outlet. It seems that weight-loss maintenance is better with Roux-en-y gastric bypass, but mainly because of diarrhoea if patients attempt to overeat again. Formal comparisons have not been conducted.

chapter 10

Establishing and running a weight-management service

To provide a professional weight-management service that is effective and sustainable, new structural developments are required. Over many years, a large body of science has become available, demonstrating the superiority of certain principles. This evidence is reviewed in the SIGN clinical guidelines[22] and forms the basis of this book. Hitherto, little attempt has been made to marshal this evidence and to apply the effective principles in a routine service setting. To some extent, most of this failure can be attributed to the generally inappropriate perceptions and goals of treatment. *It has taken very recent research to make it clear that goals of 5–10 kg weight loss, which are frequently attainable by diet and lifestyle modifications, confer major health benefits without the need to reach an ideal weight or a BMI in the normal range.*[33] To a considerable extent, this altered view (or shifted goalposts) is the result of doctors beginning to listen to their patients, and realizing that many symptoms and complications improve, and health care costs are reduced, before any distant conventional hard end points, e.g. myocardial infarction or death, can be shown to improve. The link between obesity and cardiovascular disease is real but remote, and has dominated thinking inappropriately.

In a primary care setting, it is likely that a nurse trained in weight management will usually be the firstline member of staff running a weight-management programme. A dietitian would, in theory, be the best-trained individual to run this type of programme, but in many countries there are simply not sufficient dietitians to cope with the anticipated need. For this reason, the dietitian's role in many areas will be to train other individuals, such as practice nurses, in the principles of weight management, perhaps in a rolling programme of in-service training.

Professional management and training for weight management

Consistent advice must be given by all members of the primary care team. Specific training, which might be provided by imported experts including a dietitian, a physiotherapist and a psychologist, needs to ensure up-to-date and consistent understanding of the principles and practical aspects of:

* Diet composition and nutrition
* Eating behaviour counselling
* Exercise and physical activity
* Pharmacological therapies
* Audit of results.

It is valuable to ensure that messages reaching patients from other sources are also consistent. The team should be seen to practise what it preaches. For example, coffee breaks for staff should be opportunities to take a few minutes of physical activity and, as a matter of policy, fruit rather than biscuits should be prominent at staff meetings. Educational and promotional literature in primary care centres should be scrutinized for conflicting or misleading messages. A practice weight-management team is likely to find support from other groups in the community who recognize the problem, and who would like to see rational and consistent messages transmitted clearly. Approaches from weight-management teams to local pharmacies, libraries, schools, sports facilities, journalists, cookery classes, women's groups, etc., may all provide opportunities to engage and train people with influence.

As well as having access to specialist health professionals (dietitian, physiotherapist and psychologist) for training and local planning of services, it is necessary to have standards set or negotiated, and to have a point of reference from which to judge the results of audit. Within the field of obesity and weight management, there is, as yet, no major organization bringing together the interests of patients and health professionals along the lines of the model of diabetes associations that are found in most countries. There are, however, small groups of doctors active in weight management in most countries who are in a position to establish advisory groups, to set standards in management, to coordinate research, and to work together with health promotion agencies on health education and preventive aspects of obesity. One of the challenges of the next few years is to establish the level of input necessary to control the rising figures for obesity and its attendant complications, and to justify the diversion of resources for its management.

Overweight has ubiquitous manifestations and impinges on every aspect of life. The number of potential patients is astronomical if every individual with a BMI >25 kg/m^2 is considered to be a potential patient (although the proportion with an uncontrolled weight problem and who are willing to accept help is much lower). Its management must be multidisciplinary and requires consistent messages from different professions. There is, therefore, a need for training in weight management, and often a need to enlist lay support.

Components of weight-management strategy

Risk-factor management: smoking, alcohol, blood pressure, lipids, glucose

In recognizing the seriousness of the interactions of these risk factors with risks through being overweight *(Figure 15)*, it is very important that other factors that may make things even worse are known about and dealt with. Doctors should be very clear in advising overweight patients to become non-smokers as a priority, even before moving on to deal with body weight. Blood pressure, blood cholesterol (if elevated, HDL and triglyceride in a fasting sample) and urinalysis for glucose (if positive, fasting blood glucose) should be checked. Since it is difficult to identify overweight alcohol drinkers, gamma glutamyl transferase should be checked, but it may be elevated in untreated NIDDM with fatty livers. *Specific guidance about drinking will need to be followed before weight management can be effective. This often leads to weight loss, since overweight drinkers often obtain a high calorie intake from alcohol.*

Recruiting adults in need of weight management using waist circumference action levels

Because BMI is a complicated factor, and difficult for most patients to understand or calculate, and since fat distribution is also critical in determining health risk, action levels of waist circumference (which reflect both high BMI and central fat distribution) have been proposed. Above a waist circumference of 80 cm (32 in) for women and 94 cm (37 in) for men, risks start to increase, and patients enter an 'alert' category when further increases in waist or weight should be avoided. If the waist reaches a circumference >88 cm (35 in) for women or >102 cm (40 in) for men, they enter a very-high-risk action category, where medical help should be sought and weight loss is required. These simple criteria can be employed for health promotion in a primary care setting or in the wider community. They have been adopted by the British Heart Foundation, British Diabetic Association (now called Diabetes UK) and by the Health Education Board for Scotland.

The new proactive approach to prevent weight gain needs to involve doctors and other staff offering weight-management advice routinely to normal-weight patients in a variety of situations. These include patients who need to start drugs which cause weight gain *(Table 4)*, patients who become inactive through injury and patients with family histories of weight gain at critical times such as marriage or after childbirth. A regular waist measurement check is probably valuable as a risk factor monitor.

The family

Although obesity often runs in families this is not always the case, and although husbands and wives often share physical characteristics of body composition, major changes may occur in one partner and not the other. There is a potential problem if one person in the family has a weight problem and tries to make radical changes in their diet or lifestyle. On the other hand, the dietary and lifestyle changes will bring benefits to all members of the family, whether or not they are overweight. Since the main emphasis nowadays is on *weight maintenance* and not on *weight loss*, this is also applicable to other members of the family. In the past the problem was of one individual 'going on a diet' and sometime later 'coming off a diet'. Modern advice concentrates on a healthy balanced diet and a lifestyle appropriate for everybody. Because many of the end results of poor diet and lifestyle, including obesity, are partly genetic, it is important for the future health of today's children to adopt a lifestyle and pattern of eating that will minimize long-term risks. Because everybody is tending to get fatter, people who find they have a weight problem have an important responsibility to help protect their children.

In overweight children there are very rarely grounds for advising weight loss. Risks of provoking anorexia nervosa are greater and nutritional differences could impair growth or development. On the other hand, weight management, usually to limit weight gain until the child has grown, is appropriate on a family basis.

Box 5 Criteria for evaluating a weight-management service.

- Trained staff (externally-validated training)
- Printed programme of methods
- Calibrated, maintained equipment
- Appropriate goals
- Documentation of progress and audit of outcome measures, e.g. weight risk factors
- Follow-up process defined
- Communication with general practitioner

chapter 11

Medical and health service costs of obesity and its management

The burden on medical and health services of overweight and obesity incorporates the costs in terms of direct management of the disease, and also the costs of managing secondary complications. Various analyses have been conducted in different countries to examine these costs. In general, the expenditure on management of obesity by health services is extremely small and is only a very small fraction of the total expenditure on weight management if the spending by general public on special formulated slimming foods, slimming clubs, slimming magazines, exercise bicycles, etc., is included. In the UK, the total slimming industry is worth of the order of £1–2 billion per annum. The medical management of obesity, mainly in the hands of dietitians in the National Health Service, is of the order of £1 million. There is no good estimate of the money spent by individuals on private medical care or on drugs from private sources. The cost of surgery, although relatively expensive (£1000–2000 per case), is trivially small at a national level because of the very low numbers being treated surgically.

The biggest costs of obesity for national health services are undoubtedly those of the secondary complications, and particularly the drug bills for long-term treatment of NIDDM, hyperlipidaemia, hypertension, arthritis and depression, to which must be added the costs of drugs for treating ischaemic heart disease and other conditions later in life. Obese people who develop these secondary conditions also have appreciably increased needs for medical consultation, both in primary care and in medical out-patient clinics; they also have increased and prolonged hospital in-patient stays. The overall costs of weight management in health services have been estimated at between 1 and 7% of total health care budgets, depending on the methods of analyses used. Some of the higher estimates have resulted from analyses that tended to add up the costs of treating these conditions for everybody who is overweight, without considering the background level of costs that would be present in those individuals had they not been overweight. If the method of population-attributable risk is employed, then lower estimates are made. However, the lower figures that are attained by this method are still comparable to the costs of managing other major diseases such as hypertension, diabetes and cancers *(Table 17)*.

The medical and health service costs of obesity aside, there are enormous social costs. These arise from psychological alterations in overweight people, not least because of the discrimination suffered in almost every walk of life. The depression and domestic tensions created by obesity are very substantial. Employment becomes problematic at BMI of >40 kg/m^2; unemployment is common and many specific jobs present

Table 17 Summary of cost-of-illness studies in the UK. (Reproduced with permission from Hughes and McGuire[34] and Hughes et al.[35])

Disease	*Total direct cost (£m, 1995 prices)*
Alzheimer's disease	1761
Stroke	949
Coronary heart disease	757
Diabetes	748
Obesity	355
Epilepsy	156
IDDM	108
Benign prostatic hyperplasia	104
Multiple sclerosis	41
Migraine	31

hazards for those whose BMI rises > 30 kg/m^2. Within the range of symptoms experienced by people who are overweight, many obstacles to normal employment arise. Just as one example, the increased back pain suffered by overweight people can be directly related to the time taken off work and to unemployment *(Table 9)*. Certain jobs are not available to people who are overweight because physical fitness is required, e.g. the fire service. Other jobs may not exclude the overweight as a matter of policy, but discrimination prevents the appointment of overweight individuals, e.g. in clothing and fashion shops.

Overweight people look more like older individuals. While this may have some temporary advantage for overweight young men, it is generally an impediment to social and domestic well-being. The children of very obese parents are often ashamed to be seen with them and this has an obviously divisive effect within families.

There is no doubt that proposed guidelines for comprehensive weight management in the population will substantially increase the direct costs of obesity management. In order to make this form of management possible, it will be necessary to budget strategically, recognizing that the savings that will be made within health services as a result of effective management will not be felt for a number of years. This form of strategy requires a recognition that improvement in quality of life, related to domestic and social situations, must form part of the equation. Arguing the issues on the specific case of overweight and obesity is similar to the principles that need to be addressed when deciding to implement a national health service of any kind. The greatest benefit of an effective weight management policy is likely to be felt by less able and more deprived sectors of the population.

chapter 12

Epidemic control: the quest for primary prevention

The WHO has recognized that obesity is now a global epidemic and, as such, demands efforts at prevention.[36] One of the most tantalizing aspects of obesity and weight management is its very preventability. The simplistic assertion that obesity is theoretically preventable and therefore resources should not be put into its treatment is one of the destructive arguments that have contributed to the perceived failure of medical management in recent years. On the other hand, there is as yet no established programme that has been found to be effective in the prevention of obesity or primary prevention of weight gain in susceptible individuals. There is reasonably consistent evidence that switching from a typical high-fat Western diet to a much lower fat intake will abolish or limit adult weight gain, but the threshold level may be as low as 20% energy from fat. There is also evidence that regular physical activity is the most effective way to avoid weight regain after slimming, and strong suggestions that physical activity above a certain threshold will prevent weight gain *(Box 6)*. More specifically, it is possible, from a knowledge of family histories and other predictive information, to identify young people who are at greatly increased risks of developing specific obesity-related conditions such as NIDDM. It is not the current priority within the principles of medical management for those conditions (NIDDM, ischaemic heart disease, hypertension and hyperlipidaemia) to propose weight management for young relatives of affected individuals or others. However, this may change as more comprehensive health strategies

Box 6 Benefits of physical activity.

Opposes:
- Weight gain
- Excess appetite
- Central fat deposition
- High cholestorol
- High triglyceride/low low-density lipoproteins
- Diabetes
- Hypertension
- Heart disease/stroke
- Bowel cancer
- Depression
- Osteoporosis
- Falls/fractured hips

develop and when specific research projects have produced clear evidence for the value of primary preventive intervention.

At this stage, it can reasonably be proposed that offspring of overweight parents should be the first targeted for primary preventive interventions *(Figure 29)*. The likelihood of obesity developing is *c.* 70% for those with one affected parent, increasing to nearly 90% if both parents are obese. Obviously, the number of young people who would fit these criteria would be very high and the only feasible approach could be health promotion directed at the entire population. It is worth noting that BMI tracks closely with age from late teens. So school leavers with BMI ≥ 25 kg/m^2 are highly likely (80% certainty) to have BMI ≥ 30 at age 35. This offers a focus for health promotion.

It would, however, also be reasonable to offer a more focused intervention for those whose family histories also include obesity-related diseases like NIDDM, hyperlipidaemia, ischaemic heart disease or arthritis. The type of management might involve group approaches directed towards weight maintenance, just as are proposed for the long-term management of people with proven weight problems.

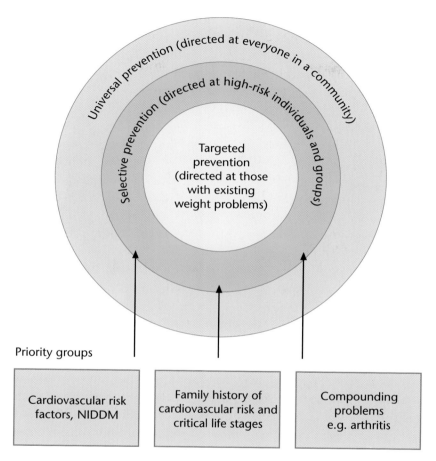

Figure 29 *Levels of prevention measures.*

The potential role of the food industry in the prevention of obesity is already a topic of general discussion. Especially formulated low-calorie versions of common foods are now available in virtually every food outlet and, in some instances, the low-calorie versions are outselling the conventional high-calorie ones, e.g. reduced-fat milk and diet-cola drinks. At present, it is difficult to establish whether this type of food development has had any impact on the rising rates of obesity. A popular view is that the availability of these products has simply meant that people consume more, or consume them in addition to their existing diet. This is an area in which there is considerable lack of good information, and this has led to widespread confusion amongst the general public and health professionals alike. As a general principle, the consumer will usually compensate, at least over a period of time, for deficits in energy intake, so people with weight problems will probably still need to restrict food intake consciously.

As with other areas of lifestyle-related health and ill health, the primary prevention of obesity is only likely to become a reality if government policies are brought together across a range of fields with the common aim of improving health and, in this context, promoting energy balance. Therefore, it will probably be necessary for the Ministries and Government Departments for Food, Agriculture, Fisheries, (including the Food Standards Agency), Trade and Industry, and Health to get together to decide the preferred compositions and promotions of foods. The marketing of foods might ideally be regulated in such as way that undesirable dietary imbalances are not promoted to susceptible and vulnerable groups, e.g. the promotion on television of high-sugar and high-saturated-fat foods to young children. Similarly, the promotion of physical activity or active living cannot rest entirely within the policies of the Government Agencies responsible for culture, media and sport, but also needs to be consistent with policies within Schools and Education, Roads, Transport, Town Planning, and Environment. Health-related messages have, for many years, recommended increased levels of physical activity, which will have benefits in many ways. Consistent policy is required to check the decline in resources for sports and recreation in schools, and to reverse the movements towards less-safe roads and environments for cycling and walking. Moves to encourage people to avoid energy-saving devices, such as escalators, lifts and elevators, motor transport for short journeys, etc., need to be endorsed and publicized, and then facilitated on a substantial basis.

One of the biggest problems facing any moves towards primary prevention of obesity in Western countries at present is the remarkable reversal in the social class profile of obesity. This is now a disease that marks deprivation and a low social class, for a variety of reasons as discussed in Chapter 3. It is difficult to see any effective programme for obesity prevention being developed in a context where the gap between the highest and lowest social classes is widening. There is some evidence that the increase in prevalence of obesity is less in countries where there is a narrower social divide within society, e.g. Finland and the Netherlands, than in countries with very wide social divides, e.g. the USA and the UK.

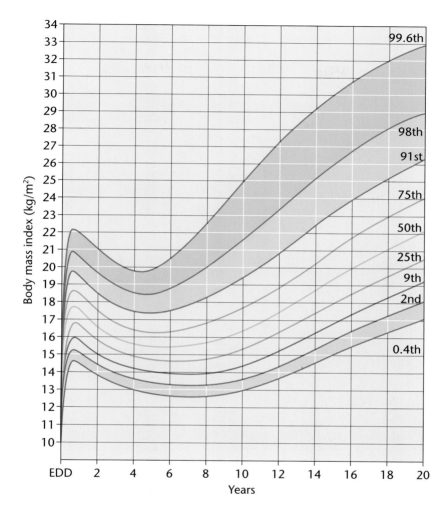

Appendix A *Male BMI chart (birth – 20 years) for the UK. © Child Growth Foundation. Reproduced with permission of the Child Growth Foundation, 2 Mayfield Avenue, Chiswick, London W4 1PW.*

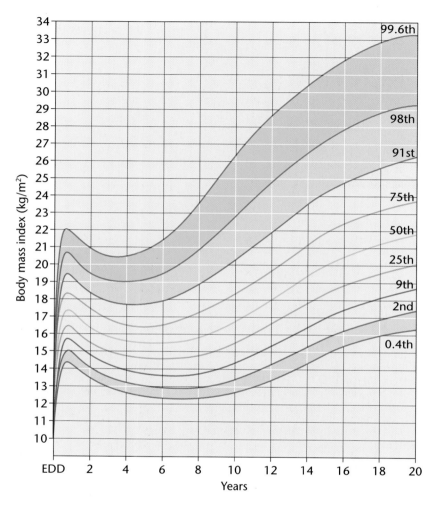

Appendix B Female BMI chart (birth – 20 years) for the UK. © Child Growth Foundation. Reproduced with permission of the Child Growth Foundation, 2 Mayfield Avenue, Chiswick, London W4 1PW.

References

1. Royal College of Physicians. Obesity. A report of the Royal College of Physicians. *J R Coll Physicians Lond* (1983) **17**: 5–65.
2. Manson JE, Willet WC, Stampfer MJ, et al. Body weight and mortality among women. *N Engl J Med* (1995) **333**: 677–85.
3. Seidell JC, Hautvast JG, Deurenberg P. Overweight: fat distribution and health risks. Epidemiological observations. A review. *Infusiontherapie* (1989) **16**: 276–81.
4. Seidell JC, Flegal KM. Assessing obesity: classification and epidemiology. *Br Med Bull* (1997) **53**: 238–52.
5. Mayer J, Thomas DW. Regulation of food intake and obesity. *Science* (1967) **156**: 328–37.
6. Han TS, van Leer EM, Seidell JC, Lean ME. Waist circumference as a screening tool for cardiovascular risk factors: evaluation of receiver operating characteristics (ROC). *Obesity Res* (1996) **4**: 533–47.
7. Department of Health. *The health of the nation. Obesity: reversing the increasing problem of obesity in England.* London: HMSO, 1995.
8. Han TS, Schouten JSAG, Lean MEJ, Seidell JC. The prevalence of low back pain and associations with body fatness, fat distribution and height. *Int J Obesity* (1997) **21**: 600–7.
9. Bump RC, Sugerman HJ, Fantl JA, et al. Obesity and lower urinary tract function in women: effect of surgically induced weight loss. *Am J Obstet Gynecol* (1992) **167**: 392–7.
10. Manson JE, Colditz GA, Meir J, et al. A prospective study of obesity and risk of coronary heart disease in women. *N Engl J Med* (1990) **322**: 882–9.
11. Chan JM, Rimm EB, Colditz GA, et al. Obesity, fat distribution, and weight gain as risk factors for clinical diabetes in men. *Diabetes Care* (1994) **17**: 961–9.
12. Colditz GA, Willet WC, Rotnitzky A, Manson JE. Weight gain as a risk factor for clinical diabetes. *Ann Int Med* (1995) **122**: 481–6.
13. Kannel WB, Brand N, Skinner JJ Jr, Dawber TR, McNamara PM. The relation of adiposity to blood pressure and development of hypertension. The Framlington Study. *Ann Intern Med* (1967) **67**: 48–59.

14. Lindroos AK, Lissner L, Sjostrom L. Weight change in relation to intake of sugar and sweet foods before and after weight reducing gastric surgery. *Int J Obes Relat Metab Disord* (1996) **20**: 634–43.

15. Fontaine KR, Cheskin LJ, Barofsky I. Health-related quality of life in obese persons seeking treatment. *J Fam Pract* (1996) **43**: 265–70.

16. Diabetes Prevention Program Research Group. Reduction in the incidence of type 2 diabetes with lifestyle intervention or metformin. *N Engl J Med* (2002) **346**: 393–403.

17. Sjostrom L, Torgerson JS, Hauptman J, Boldrin M. XENDOS (Xentical in the prevention of diabetes in obese subjects): a landmark study. (2002) (unpublished) http://www.pslgroup.com/dg/21c116.htm

18. Karlsson J, Sjostrom L, Sullivan M. Swedish Obese Subjects (SOS) – an intervention study of obesity. Two-year follow-up of health-related quality of life (HRQL) and eating behavior after gastric surgery for severe obesity. *Int J Obes Metab Disord* (1998) **22**: 113–26.

19. Lean ME, Powrie JK, Anderson AS, et al. Obesity, weight loss and prognosis in type 2 diabetes. *Diabet Med* (1990) **7**: 228–33.

20. Williamson DF, Pamuk E, Thun M, et al. Prospective study of intentional weight loss and mortality in never-smoking overweight US white women aged 40–64. *Am J Epidemiol* (1995) **141**: 1128–41.

21. National Institutes of Health, National Heart Lung and Blood Institute. Clinical guidelines on the identification, evaluation and treatment of overweight and obesity in adults – the evidence report (1998) (http://www.nhlbi.nih.gov/guidelines/obesity/ob_home.htm).

22. Scottish Intercollegiate Guidelines Network (SIGN). Obesity in Scotland: integrating prevention with weight management (SIGN: 1996) (http://www.show.scot.nhs.uk/sign/guidelines)

23. Westrate JA, van het Hof KH, van den Berg H, et al. A comparison of the effect of free access to reduced fat products or their full fat equivalents on food intake, body weight, blood lipids and fat-soluble antioxidants levels and haemostasis variables. *EJCN* (1998) **52**: 389–95.

24. Schofield WN, Schofield C, James WPT. Basal metabolic rate: review and prediction, together with annotated bibliography of source material. *Hum Nutr: Appl Nutr* (1985) **39C**: 5–96.

25. Scottish Intercollegiate Guidelines Network (SIGN). Intercollegiate Guidelines Network: Obesity in Scotland: Integrating Prevention with Weight Management. SIGN (1996). www.show.scot.nhs.uk/sign/guidelines

26. Epstein LH, Valoski A, Wing RR, et al. Ten-year outcomes of behavioral family-based treatment for childhood obesity. *Health Psychol* (1994) **13**: 373–83.

27. Prochasta JO, DiClemente CC. Stages of change in the modification of problem behaviours. *Prog Behaviour Modification* (1992) **28**: 183–218.

28. Fishbein M, Ajzen I. Belief, attitude, intention and behaviour: an introduction to theory and research. Reading: Addison Wesley MA, 1975.

29. Saris WH. Physical inactivity and metabolic factors as predictors of weight gain. *Nutr Rev* (1996) **54**: 110–15.

30. James WPT, Astrup A, Finer N, et al. Effect of sibutramine on weight maintenance after weight loss: a randomised trial. *Lancet* (2000) **356**: S2119–25.

31. Royal College of Physicians. *Clinical management of overweight and obese patients. A report of a working party of RCP.* London: RCP, 1998.
32. Agren G, Narbro K, Naslund I, et al. Long-term effects of weight loss on pharmaceutical costs in obese subjects. A report from the SOS intervention study. *Int J Obesity* (2002) **26**: 184–92.
33. Goldstein D. Beneficial health effects of modest weight loss. *Int J Obes Relat Metab Disord* (1992) **16**: 397–415.
34. Hughes D, McGuire A. A review of the economic analysis of obesity. *Br Med Bull* (1997) **53**: 253–63.
35. Hughes D, McGuire A, Elliot H, et al. The cost of obesity in the United Kingdom. *J Med Econ* (1999) **2**: 143–53.
36. WHO. Obesity: Preventing and managing the global epidemic. WHO report of a consultation on obesity, Geneva 3–5 June (1997).

Further reading

Colditz GA. Economic costs of obesity. *Am J Clin Nutr* (1992) **55** (suppl 2): 503s–507s.

Institute of Medicine. Weighing the options. Criteria for evaluation weight management programs (PR Thomas, ed). National Academic Press: Washington DC, 1995.

Lean MEJ, Han TS, Seidell JC. Impairment of health and quality of life in people with large waist circumference. *Lancet* (1988) **351**: 853–6.

Levy E, Levy P, Le Pen C, et al. The economic cost of obesity: the French situation. *Int J Obes Relat Metab Disord* (1995) **19**: 788–92.

Seidell JC. The impact of obesity on health status: some implications for health care costs. *Int J Obes Relat Metab Disord* (1995) **19** (suppl 6): s13–s16.

Index